Acquired Language Disorders

A CASE-BASED APPROACH

Acquired Language Disorders
A CASE-BASED APPROACH

Evelyn R. Klein, Ph.D., CCC-SLP
James M. Mancinelli, M.S., CCC-SLP

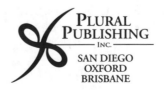

PLURAL
PUBLISHING
INC.

SAN DIEGO
OXFORD
BRISBANE

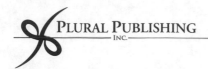

5521 Ruffin Road
San Diego, CA 92123

e-mail: info@pluralpublishing.com
Web site: http://www.pluralpublishing.com

49 Bath Street
Abingdon, Oxfordshire OX14 1EA
United Kingdom

FSC

Mixed Sources

Product group from well-managed
forests and other controlled sources

Cert no. SW-COC-002283
www.fsc.org
© 1996 Forest Stewardship Council

Typeset in 10½/13 Garamond book by Flanagan's Publishing Services, Inc.
Printed in the United States of America by McNaughton & Gunn, Inc.
Second printing, March 2010

Library of Congress Cataloging-in-Publication Data

Klein, Evelyn R.
  Acquired language disorders : a case-based approach / Evelyn R. Klein and James M. Mancinelli.
    p. ; cm.
  Includes bibliographical references and index.
  ISBN-13: 978-1-59756-055-9 (alk. paper)
  ISBN-10: 1-59756-055-3 (alk. paper)
   1. Language disorders—Case studies. 2. Aphasia—Case studies. I. Mancinelli, James M. II. Title.
   [DNLM: 1. Language Disorders—diagnosis—Problems and Exercises. 2. Aphasia—diagnosis—Problems and Exercises. 3. Aphasia—therapy—Problems and Exercises. 4. Language Disorders—therapy—Problems and Exercises. 5. Language Therapy—Problems and Exercises. WL 18.2 K64a 2009]
  RC423.K555 2009
  616.85'5—dc22

                                                              2009017447

Contents

Accompanying PowerPoint slides and CD include lecture material for Chapters 1 through 9 in this book.

Preface

Introduction

Integrating theoretical knowledge into clinical practice is challenging for new and experienced clinicians alike. Until a clinician actually encounters a person with a specific disorder, academic knowledge may remain disconnected and amorphous. It is our intention as practitioners and educators to bridge the gap between theory and practice by providing the reader with a case-based approach to understanding acquired language disorders (ALD). To further our goal in making ALD come to life for the reader, we have developed a diagram that depicts the individual's language and cognition following a CVA or other neurologic event. We refer to this as the Acquired Language Disorders Target Model (ALD Target Model) and each of the 14 cases that we discuss has a corresponding diagram (see Appendix D). In our experience at the graduate level, the student benefits from the graphic features of the ALD Target Model because it facilitates a concrete understanding of the case and characteristics of the disorder. This model combined with characteristics of the various disorders, case analyses, and treatment considerations connects theoretical knowledge with practical application. In our opinion, this case-based approach matches the needs of speech-language pathologists practicing in health care today.

How the Book Is Organized

We decided to apply the case-based approach to the topic by building each chapter around a fictional person, based on a real case, exemplifying a specific acquired language disorder. This brings the communication impairment to life for the learner who can now conceptualize the specific characteristics of the disorder in the context of a real person. These case scenarios were developed based on actual patients who the authors or their colleagues have evaluated and treated. For purposes of anonymity and confidentiality, the patients' names and identifying information have been changed. As practicing speech-language pathologists we believe it is essential to understand not only the basic pathophysiology of a disease process associated with an acquired language disorder, but also the functional effects it may have on a person's life. It is not our intention to provide the reader with detailed and comprehensive knowledge of neurologic disease, but we do provide the basic neurologic features of the disorders discussed. The fundamentals presented here will allow the reader to participate in discussions with other professionals and family members. The student or practitioner can then use this information to build a foundation for assessment and therapeutic approaches, many of which are found in Appendix E.

Special Features

The 14 cases in this book provide a comprehensive overview of the assessment process, major aphasic syndromes, right hemisphere disorders, traumatic brain injury, dementia, encephalopathy, and other etiologies affecting the ability to communicate. The final chapter provides detailed information on therapeutic approaches currently in use, and includes future trends in treatment along with a discussion about evidence-based practice.

Each chapter based on a case study includes eight sections:

- **Characteristics** of the disorder including neurologic correlates
- **Case Scenario** providing past medical and social history

- **Diagnostic Profile** including language expression, speech, auditory comprehension, reading, written expression, cognition, and behavioral symptoms
- The **ALD Target Model** graphically represents language and cognitive features of each case
- **Functional Analysis** consists of a narrative that succinctly summarizes the case and helps the clinician understand the impact of this disability on the patient's daily life.
- **Critical Thinking/Learning Activity** poses questions designed to develop problem-solving and practical skills necessary to maximize the patient's progress.
- **Treatment Considerations** provide areas to consider for rehabilitation, as well as general therapeutic objectives
- **Therapeutic Options** pertinent to the cases are listed and further described in Appendix E.

The Acquired Language Disorders Target Model

We developed the Acquired Language Disorders Target Model (ALD Target Model) from an *embedded language framework*. This model is shown in Figure 1 and reflects the influence that cognition plays in normal communication and, by extension, in the rehabilitation of people with acquired language disorders. The physical appearance of the model depicts the relationship between language and cognition as well as the relationship among functional language modalities. The components of communication, Expression (E), Comprehension (C), Reading (R), and Writing (W), form the *language complex*. Reading, part of the Visual modality, and Writing (including drawing) part of the Graphic modality, are located on the horizontal axis. Comprehension (C) includes comprehension of verbal and gestural language and Expression (E) includes verbal and gestural expression located on the vertical axis of the diagram.

Normal Communication Embedded within Normal Cognitive Functions

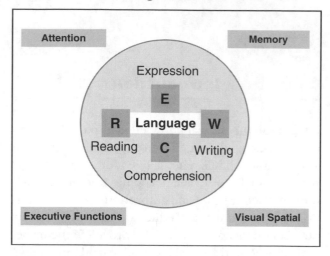

Figure 1. The Acquired Language Disorders Target Model.

For an individual who has normal communication functions, the lettered squares (E, C, R, and W) remain attached to the word "Language." For an individual with an acquired language disorder, the lettered squares move further away from the central position to reflect the severity of impairment. For each type of acquired language disorder, the pattern is different. For example, in a person with an expressive nonfluent aphasia (Broca's), the E square and the W square are moved outside the circular border to indicate a severe degree of impairment. Depending on the acquired language disorder, any or all of these language modality areas may be impaired. This ranges from normal, to mild-moderate, to moderate-severe, to severe-profound. This is depicted in Figure 2.

The ALD Target Model supports the cognitive domains of Helm-Estabrooks and Albert (2004) and illustrates cognitive deficits. The domains are attention, memory, visuospatial, and executive functions, which are described in Chapter 2. The reader will notice a fracture through any of the four cognitive domains that are impaired. For example, in an individual with a severely impaired memory, the box labeled memory depicts this fracture.

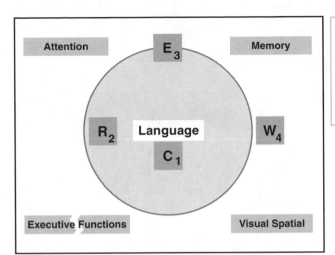

Figure 2. The key to understanding the Acquired Language Disorders Target Model.

How to Use This Book

For the Student and the Practitioner

■ A graphic image of the ALD Model representing each disorder enhances the student's or practitioner's understanding of cognitive-linguistic changes pertinent to the case. The reader should note that this case represents only one example of this disorder and is not representative of all.

■ Case comparisons facilitate more accurate decision-making for treatment.

■ The ALD model combined with the Functional Analysis can be very useful for clinical practice in a health care setting. This permits the student or practitioner to integrate the neurologic, cognitive, linguistic, and functional aspects of each patient to formulate a holistic picture.

■ PowerPoint slides supporting lectures are provided for Chapters 1 to 9 in the book.

■ Critical thinking questions are provided for each case to facilitate clinical decision-making skills.

■ Many current treatment approaches are provided to assist the practitioner in planning a program for each patient.

■ A one-page diagnostic profile describes each patient's language expression, speech, auditory comprehension, reading, written expression, cognition, and behavioral symptoms.

For the Instructor

■ An overview of basic neuroanatomy for acquired language disorders is provided.

■ This book offers a detailed summary of many formal and informal assessment and treatment programs.

■ There are 14 case-based acquired language disorders, each with assessment and treatment considerations, to facilitate class discussion and clinical problem-solving.

■ There is a section on evidence-based practice from an historical perspective.

■ PowerPoint slides for Chapters 1 to 9 correspond with the text and offer lecture material.

■ Charts, tables, and figures including the ALD Target Model help categorize and concretize the various acquired language disorders.

Reference

Helm-Estabrooks, N., & Albert, M. L. (2004). *Manual of aphasia and aphasia therapy* (2nd ed.). Austin, TX: Pro-Ed.

Acknowledgments

Writing a book requires not only dedication and knowledge from the authors but also the support and involvement of other people. We would like to acknowledge the work of Ami Van Dine, and Erin Hayes, two dedicated graduate students in the Speech-Language-Hearing Science Program at La Salle University, who provided invaluable support. We also acknowledge the fine work of our illustrator, Brain Nugent, whose attention to detail is greatly appreciated. As university professors, we are grateful for the interest from our program director, Dr. Barbara Amster, whose encouragement and support helped us throughout the process. In addition, we are fortunate to have had the guidance and excellent input from our editor, Stephanie Meissner, and our production assistant, Lauren Narasky, who were always available and willing to assist us. Thank you! Finally, we want to thank the staff at Plural Publishing who saw the value of this project and facilitated its completion.

Jim Mancinelli would like to thank his colleague and co-author, Evelyn Klein, for her patience, trust, intellect, and her astounding ability to make him smile. It was an honor and a pleasure to work with her on this book. As always, Mr. Mancinelli must acknowledge a very special Squirrel, whose love and understanding sustained him during this project. Thanks, SB!

Evelyn Klein would like to thank Jim Mancinelli for joining her in this project. His ideas in the formation of this text are what make it unique. Working with Jim on this book was never a task; it was an interesting and informative joining of experience and knowledge. She is eternally grateful that he took the plunge!

Brian Nugent, the illustrator for this book, has a portfolio that can be viewed at www.sktnrd.com .

About the Authors

Evelyn R. Klein,
Ph.D., CCC-SLP/L, BRS-CL

Dr. Evelyn R. Klein is Associate Professor of Speech-Language-Hearing Science at La Salle University in Philadelphia, Pennsylvania. She is a licensed and certified speech-language pathologist and licensed psychologist with postdoctoral training in neuropsychology. She holds Board Specialty Recognition in Child Language from the American Speech-Language-Hearing Association and has Supervisory Certification in Special Education from the Pennsylvania Department of Education. Dr. Klein maintains an active private practice.

Dr. Klein is a teacher, clinician, and researcher. She teaches, supervises, and advises undergraduate and graduate students pursuing a degree in speech-language pathology. Her areas of specialization include language-learning disabilities, acquired language disorders, research design, and counseling for communicative disorders. For more than 25 years she has evaluated and treated children, teens, and adults with communication disorders in rehabilitation facilities, schools, and private practice with a focus on cognitive neuropsychology and language disorders.

As a researcher and author, Dr. Klein has co-developed *Focus On Function* (2nd ed.) and *Focus On Transition*, two therapeutic programs for individuals with aphasia and cognitive-linguistic deficits. She is also the coauthor of the *Hear It, Say It, Learn It*, a new program for literacy. Dr. Klein currently is conducting research about symbol learning and visual-verbal associations related to working memory. Other areas of investigation include assessment models for evaluating speech and language skills in children with selective mutism.

Dr. Klein mentors undergraduate and graduate students in the pursuit of their own research interests. She continues to publish in peer-reviewed journals and presents her work at local, national, and international conferences.

James M. Mancinelli,
M.S. CCC-SLP/L

James M. Mancinelli is the University Clinical Coordinator in the Speech-Language-Hearing Science Program in the School of Nursing and Health Sciences at La Salle University in Philadelphia, Pennsylvania. He is a licensed and certified speech-language pathologist.

Mr. Mancinelli is a teacher, administrator, clinician, and researcher. At La Salle University he advises graduate students pursuing a masters degree in speech-language pathology, teaches undergraduate courses, graduate level clinical practicum, and the medical speech pathology elective. As an administrator, he is responsible for developing relationships with external affiliates, establishing clinical contracts, and arranging for clinical externships.

He has 25 years of clinical experience in medical speech-language pathology, and is clinically active within the Crozer-Keystone Health System in Upland, Pennsylvania. His focus has always been neurogenic communication and swallowing disorders. He has worked in acute care, acute rehab, subacute rehab, and long-term care, as well as outpatient therapy with adults with neurogenic communication and voice disorders. His research interests include acquired apraxia of speech, neurogenic communication disorders, and clinical education. Mr. Mancinelli has published work on ALS and has presented both at the Cleveland Clinic and at ASHA. He considers it an honor to be able to work with the staff and faculty in the SLHS Program at La Salle University.

Jim Mancinelli dedicates this work to his parents, Gus and Dolores, whose love and commitment to his happiness and well-being got him to where he is today.

Evelyn Klein dedicates this book to her husband, Dietrich Franczuszki, and children Ross, Scott, Matthew, Sarina, Elisha, Marisa, and Ben, whose support, patience, and love make all the difference!

Chapter 1

AN OVERVIEW OF NEUROANATOMY AND NEUROPHYSIOLOGY RELATED TO ACQUIRED LANGUAGE DISORDERS (ALD)

The Neuron

The brain has more than 100 billion neurons, or nerve cells. These structures comprise the building blocks of the nervous system and are its functional "work horses." Each neuron is composed of a body, referred to as the soma; filamental extensions called dendrites; and longer fibers called axons. Each neuron has one axonal fiber that can measure from micrometers to meters in length. The axon functions as a conductor of electrical impulses. Dendrites receive stimuli or input from other neurons and axons send stimuli to other neurons, glands, or muscles (Webb & Adler, 2008). These neurons communicate with each other electrochemically via neurotransmitters (a discussion of neurotransmitters appears in this chapter) (Figure 1–1).

The nervous system has sensory neurons (receptors) and motor neurons (effectors). Sensory neurons are sensitive to light, sound, touch, temperature, smell, and chemical input and transmit sensory information from the environment via the nervous system. Motor neurons receive excitation from other cells and send impulses to the muscles instructing them to contract and to the endocrine glands to regulate hormonal secretions. Input from sensory

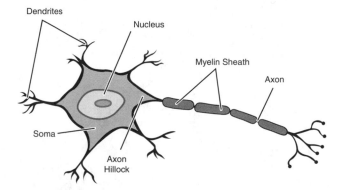

Figure 1–1. Neuron.

neurons can be transmitted to motor neurons. Interneurons comprise the largest group of neurons and connect one neuron to another. For example, a sensory neuron may detect a dangerous stimulus and respond by alerting interneurons in the spinal cord to notify the motor neurons to remove that body part in danger. At the endpoint or terminal of the nerve cell, neurotransmitters are released into the synaptic space between the cells. Neurotransmitters are biochemical compounds that help neurons communicate, acting as messengers between them (Figures 1–2 and 1–3).

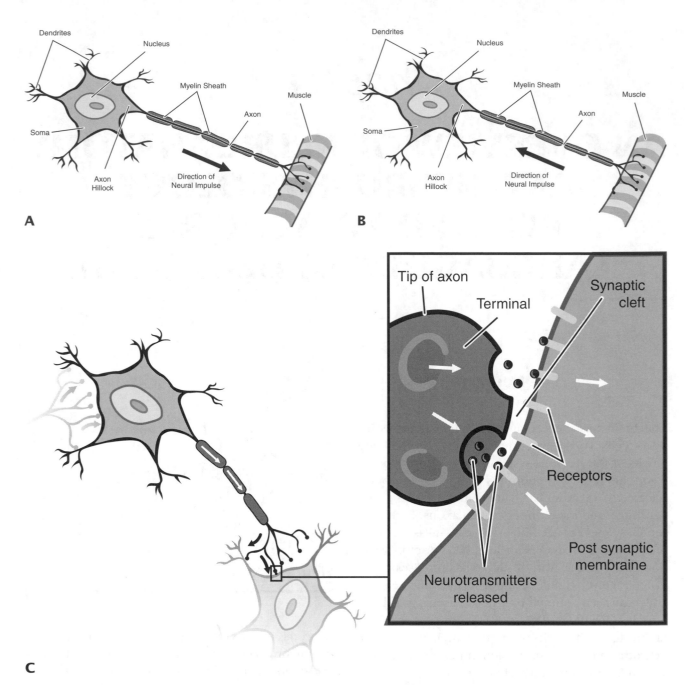

Figure 1–2. (**A**) Motor neuron, (**B**) sensory neuron, and (**C**) events at synapse.

Neurotransmitters

Neurotransmitters are chemicals that assist in the regulation of the brain's ability to control metabolic activity, speech and language, motivation, personality, mood states, and cognition including attention and memory (Bhatnagar, 2002). Each neuron releases neurotransmitters at the synapse, which is where the bulb of the axon makes contact with the dendrites. The neurotransmitter passes across the synaptic cleft and bonds with the receptor site on the post-

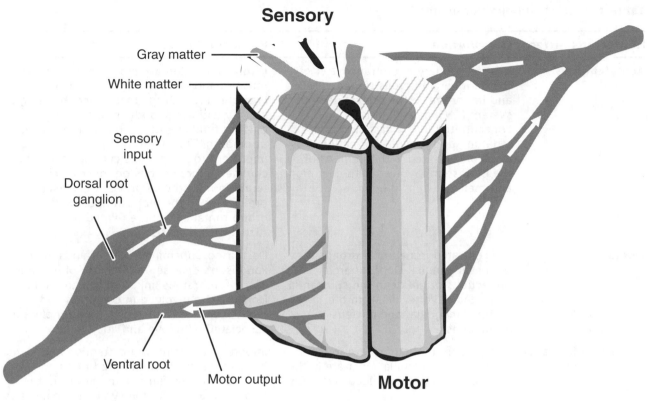

Figure 1–3. Spinal cord cross-section.

synaptic membrane. This results in a change in the electrical current across the cell membrane and the nerve fibers. The change in the electrical valence of the cell is referred to as the action potential. An excess or depletion of neurotransmitters can have significant effects on functioning. For example, excess dopamine has been linked to schizophrenia, and a depletion of dopamine concentration contributes to Parkinson's disease.

There are two main types of neurotransmitters: the small molecules and the large molecules, also known as neuropeptides. The small molecule transmitters include acetylcholine, serotonin, dopamine, norepinephrine, glutamate, histamine, and gamma aminobutyric acid (GABA). In this group, GABA is primarily inhibitory whereas glutamate is excitatory. Yet, in many cases, neurotransmitters can be either excitatory or inhibitory depending on the receptor site. Dopamine can act in this way. The large molecule neuropeptides include vasopressin, somatostatin, neurotensin, enkephalin, and endorphins. These neuroactive substances are hormone mediated and affect the body's metabolic functioning. A pituitary peptide such as endorphin is opioid-like and functions in pain management. Neuroactive peptides may be specific to particular organs and have multiple roles in the body. Both groups of neurotransmitters are crucial to a person's feelings of pleasure, pain, stress, cravings, the promotion of sleep and rest, and emotional attachment, as well as basic metabolic functioning (Webb & Adler, 2008; Schwartz, 1991) (Table 1–1).

The Brain: A Brief Review of Structure and Function

The central nervous system consists of the brain and spinal cord. Each segment of the spinal cord has both sensory and motor nerves that innervate our skin, organs, and muscles. During brain development in

Table 1-1. Selected Neurotransmitters

Neurotransmitter	Distribution	Proposed Impact
Acetylcholine	It is the primary neurotransmitter of the peripheral nervous system (PNS) and important to the central nervous system (CNS) as well. It is concentrated in the basal forebrain, striatum, and reticular formation. It is also concentrated within regions of the brainstem involved with cognition and memory.	Involved in voluntary movement of skeletal muscles and viscera including spinal and cranial nerves. Drugs that affect cholinergic activity within the body impact heart rate, bladder function, digestion, and may cause dry mouth. This neurotransmitter is also important to sleep-wake cycles. Decreased cholinergic projections on muscle cells are found in myasthenia gravis. Decreased projections in the hippocampus and orbitofrontal cortex are related to Alzheimer's disease.
Dopamine	Concentrated in neuronal groups in the basal ganglia. Dopaminergic projections originate in the substantia nigra and have terminals in the cortex, amygdala, and nucleus accumbens.	Decreased dopamine in the brain is linked to Parkinson's disease. An increase of dopamine in the forebrain is linked to schizophrenia. Dopamine is involved in cognition and motivation and is related to wanting pleasure associated with love and addiction.
Norepinephrine	Norepinephrine neurons are found in the pons and medulla. Most are in the reticular formation and locus ceruleus.	Important to maintaining attention and focus. It increases excitation in the brain and is involved in wakefulness and arousal. It is also associated with the sympathetic nervous system and feelings of panic "fight or flight."
Serotonin	Synthesized from amino acid tryptophan, found in blood platelets and gastrointestinal tract. Terminals are localized in nerve pathways from the nuclei at the center of the reticular formation.	Controls mood, regulates sleep, involved in perception of pain, body temperature, blood pressure, and hormonal functioning. Low levels are associated with depression. It is also involved in memory and emotion.
GABA	A major neurotransmitter with cells found in the cerebral cortex, cerebellum, and hippocampus. GABA projections are inhibitory from the striatum to the globus pallidus and substantia nigra to the thalamus.	Loss of GABA in the striatum is linked to a degenerative disease which causes involuntary abnormal movements (Huntington's chorea). It is associated with the inhibition of motor neurons.

childhood neurons create new connections with other neurons. At birth the brain weighs about 350 grams (12 ounces) and is about 1,000 grams (2.2 pounds) at one year old. As an adult, the brain weighs approximately 1,200 to 1,400 grams (2.6 to 3.1 pounds) and does not have the ability to create new connections with other neurons as most neurons cannot be replaced. This section discusses the brain's covering, the ventricles, and the following major structures of the central nervous system: the cerebral cortex, brainstem, subcortical structures, cerebellum, and the neural pathways.

The Coverings of the Brain, Ventricles, and Cerebrospinal Fluid

There are three layers of tissues, the meninges, that protect the brain. They include the dura mater, arachnoid membrane, and pia mater. Between the arachnoid membrane and pia mater is the subarachnoid space. This space contains blood vessels and cerebrospinal fluid (CSF).

The CSF protects the brain. It is a clear and colorless fluid that circulates throughout the brain and the spinal cord cushioning and protecting them from injury. There are four ventricles within the brain: two lateral ventricles, the third ventricle, and the fourth ventricle. Each ventricle contains the choroid plexus, which is the structure that produces the CSF. The CSF flows from one ventricle to the next and finally into the subarachnoid space. It is reabsorbed back into the blood. The lateral ventricles are connected to the third ventricle and the third ventricle is connected to the fourth. Blockage in any of the spaces can cause CSF to back up leading to a number of serious medical conditions including hydrocephalus, which increases pressure on the brain (http://www.sickkids.ca/childphysiology/cpwp/brain/csf.htm) (Figures 1-4 and 1-5).

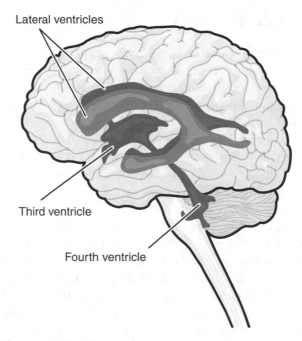

Figure 1–4. Ventricles.

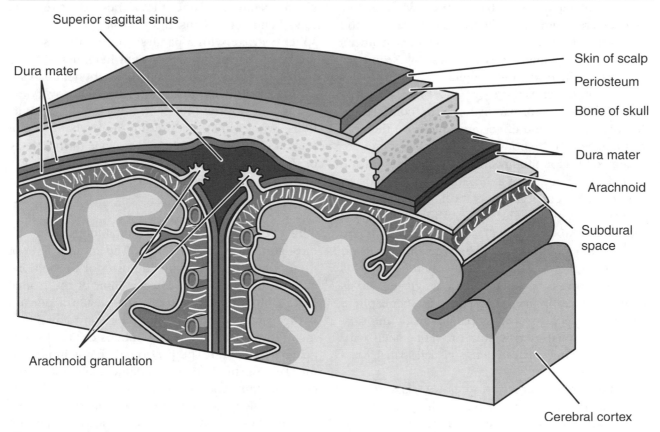

Figure 1–5. Meninges.

Cerebral Cortex

The cerebral cortex is also referred to as the cerebrum and it comprises the largest part of the brain. It is involved in complex thought, learning, personality, movement, touch, and vision and is divided into two hemispheres: right and left. The outer surface of each hemisphere is composed of gray matter that contains nerve cell bodies (more than 6 billion), glial cells, capillaries, axons, and dendrites. The gray matter directs sensory or motor stimuli to the interneurons of the central nervous system for responsiveness via synaptic activation. White matter consists of axons that travel throughout the cortex. These structures are referred to as "white matter" due to the color of the myelinated sheaths that wrap each axon. The color reflects the fact that they consist primarily of lipids, or fatty material. As noted in the section on neurons, the axon is responsible for carrying information away from the brain to the periphery. These axons form tracts and the tracts take the information to their intended destination. Two neurologic diseases that manifest white matter changes are multiple sclerosis which destroys the myelin shield surrounding the axons and Alzheimer's disease. In Alzheimer's disease these white matter changes produce amyloid plaques.

The two hemispheres of the brain primarily receive sensory information from the contralateral side of the body and effect movement on the contralateral side of the body. The two hemispheres are separated by a longitudinal fissure but communicate by two large bundles of axons, the corpus callosum composed of cortical association fibers and subcortical connections. The proper and efficient functioning of the corpus callosum is critical to the transmission of information between the left and right hemispheres. The left hemisphere typically is best for processing speech and language and is involved in verbal memory. The right hemisphere has been known to process paralinguistic information and pragmatics as well as providing skills with nonlinguistic information that is visual, spatial, emotional, and musical.

The cerebral cortex integrates sensory and motor signals in order to execute the primary sensory, motor, and association area functions.

The sensory areas pf the cortex receive input from the environment such as touch, taste, smell, vision, and hearing. The motor areas are responsible for muscular activity throughout the body. The association areas of the cortex connect the sensory and motor systems and give humans the ability to integrate the sensory (afferent) and the motor (efferent) information, permitting normal function.

The following Web site provides an overview of midsagittal brain structures and functions (Figure 1–6): http://web.psych.ualberta.ca/~iwinship/studyguide/brain_study.htm .

Lobes of the Brain

Each hemisphere is composed of four lobes: the frontal, temporal, parietal, and occipital (Figure 1–7). The left side of the brain generally controls the right side of the body and the right hemisphere controls the left side of the body. Damage to either hemisphere can result in paralysis or lost sensation. Weakness on one side of the body is referred to as hemiparesis and paralysis on one side of the body is referred to as hemiplegia. Thus, if a person has a left hemispheric stroke with a paralysis on the right side of the body, that person has a right hemiplegia. If the right side is only weak, it is then a right hemiparesis.

The following Web site provides an overview of the lobes of the brain and their associated functions: www.stanford.edu/group/hopes/basics/braintut/ab4.html . The lateral views provide further detail of the structural landmarks and functional association areas of a cerebral hemisphere (Figures 1–8A and 1–8B).

The Frontal Lobes. The frontal lobes are at the most anterior part of the brain. The anterior limit of the frontal lobe is dorsal and posterior to the bony case of the eyes. The posterior limit of the frontal lobes is the precentral gyrus. The posterior portion of the frontal lobe is specialized for control of movement. In humans, the frontal lobe is critical for language production. The prefrontal area is important for planning and initiation, judgment and reasoning, concentration, emotional range, disinhibition of behaviors, and adaptation to change. Functions of the frontal lobes are essential to consciousness and let

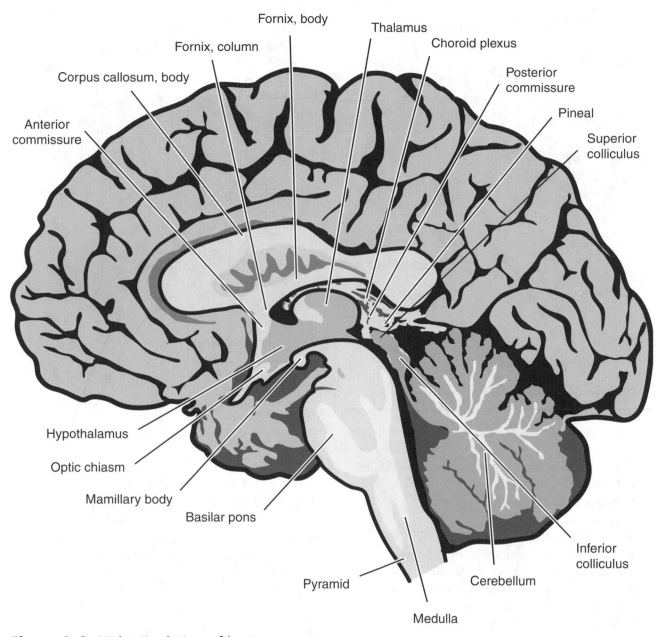

Figure 1–6. Midsagittal view of brain.

us appropriately judge what we are doing in the environment and how we initiate and respond to life's events. Proper functioning assists with our emotional response and expressive language choices. Essentially, the frontal lobes make us aware of our conscious actions. Our emotional responses, memory for habits, motor activities, and expressive language are all mediated by the frontal lobe.

People who have frontal lobe damage may have the following:

■ Loss of simple movement (paralysis)

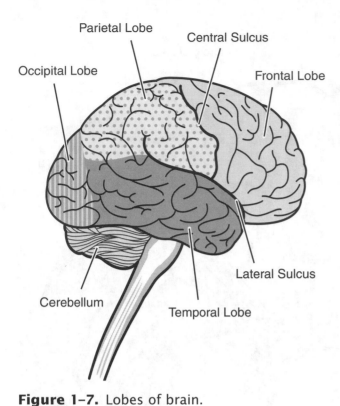

Figure 1–7. Lobes of brain.

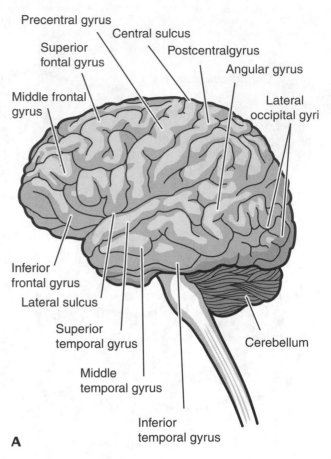

A

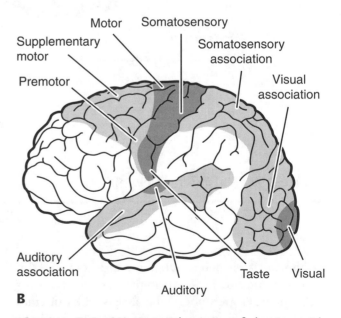

B

- Loss of spontaneously interacting with others
- Loss of flexible thinking
- Persistence on a single thought (perseveration)
- Inability to focus on a task
- Mood changes that are frequent and inappropriate (emotional lability)
- Changes in personality and social behavior
- Difficulty problem-solving
- Inability to express language (Broca's nonfluent aphasia)
- Inability to sequence complex movements

The Temporal Lobes. The temporal lobes are located laterally in the cerebral hemispheres, approximately at the level of the ears. They house the primary and secondary auditory cortex and are involved in auditory sensation and perception. Wernicke's area is located in the posterior part of the superior temporal gyrus and important to auditory comprehension of language. It is in this area that auditory stimuli are transformed for comprehension. However,

Figure 1–8. (A) Lateral view of brain with structural landmarks, and **(B)** lateral view of brain with primary functions and secondary association areas.

many associations connect auditory input with other systems including memory needed for the auditory comprehension of language. Hearing ability, some visual perceptions, and categorization skills are dependent, in part, on the temporal lobe. The left temporal lobe contains Wernicke's area which is critical to language comprehension. Damage to the temporal association cortex may lead to difficulty identifying and categorizing auditory stimuli. The main functions of the temporal lobe include hearing ability, memory acquisition, visual perceptions, and categorization of objects. Individuals who have lesions in this area may demonstrate the following:

- Difficulty in recognizing faces (prosopagnosia)
- Difficulty understanding spoken words (Wernicke's aphasia)
- Difficulty identifying and verbalizing about objects
- Disturbance with selective attention to what is seen and heard
- Short-term memory loss
- Interference with long-term memory
- Increased or decreased interest in sexual behavior
- Inability to categorize objects
- Right lobe damage can result in persistent talking
- Increased aggressive behavior
- Poor selective attention to what is seen or heard

The ability to understand written and spoken language occurs primarily in Wernicke's area and the ability to produce speech movement occurs primarily in the frontal lobe (Broca's area). These two areas communicate with each other constantly via bundles of neurons that are subcortical white matter pathways known as the arcuate fasciculus and superior longitudinal fasciculus. These pathways also pass through gyri at the rim of the sylvian fissure (angular gyrus and supramarginal gyrus) which are also very important areas for the language modalities.

The Parietal Lobes. The parietal lobes are located between the occipital lobe and the central sulcus. The most anterior part is the postcentral gyrus where the axons carrying sensory information for the sensation terminate. The parietal lobe receives and evaluates most sensory information including touch, pressure, pain, temperature, and taste. Sensations from the body are represented at various parts of the postcentral gyrus. A person with parietal lobe damage may demonstrate the following deficits:

- Inability to attend to more than one object at a point in time
- Inability to name an object (anomia)
- Problems with reading (alexia)
- Inability to write words (agraphia)
- Word blindness (inability to recognize words)
- Difficulty with math (dyscalculia)
- Difficulty drawing objects
- Difficulty knowing left from right
- Lack of awareness of specific body parts
- Inability to focus visual attention
- Difficulties with eye-hand coordination
- Impaired perception of touch
- Unilateral neglect
- Inability to manipulate objects

The Occipital Lobes. The occipital lobes are located at the posterior part of the brain. It is the primary target for projections from the thalamus and it receives sensory information from fibers in the eyes. The retina gets visual input in the form of light flashes, shapes, and shading. This input is then transmitted through the optic nerve to the thalamus and then to the primary visual cortex in the occipital lobe. If the visual cortex is damaged, blindness or a partial visual field cut can ensue. For example, damage to the left hemisphere often impairs vision in the right visual field. A small focal area of damage or lesion can lead to a small blind area or scotoma. Although the neural information is initially meaningless, the association areas of the cortex transmit stimuli to other parts of the brain for analysis. The medial and lateral surfaces of the occipital lobe help with such visual associations. This secondary area of the occipital lobe is important to visual processing for recognizing objects and visually discriminating.

Damage to the occipital lobe may include but are not limited to the following:

- Defects in vision such as visual field cuts

- Difficulty locating objects in the environment
- Difficulty recognizing drawn objects
- Inability to recognize movement of an object
- Difficulty identifying colors
- Visual illusions or inaccurately seeing objects
- Word blindness or inability to recognize words
- Difficulties with reading and writing

The Insula. This portion of the cerebrum is sometimes referred to as the fifth lobe. It cannot be seen like the other four lobes as it is in underneath the parietal, temporal, and frontal lobes, deep within the lateral fissure. The insula is considered a critical area for both sensory and motor functions and has been found to be related to speech and language skills. The connections and functions of the insula have not been fully described in the literature and await further investigation.

The Brainstem

The brainstem consists of the medulla oblongata, pons, and the midbrain (Figure 1–9). These structures are also referred to as the mesencephalon. The cerebellum may also be considered as part of the brainstem as it is located rostral to the spinal cord. However, it is discussed separately in this text.

The brainstem connects the brain to the spinal cord and regulates primary life functions such as respiration, swallowing, blood pressure, eye movements, and heart rate. It also mediates functions such as vomiting, salivation, sneezing, coughing, and gagging. Sensations from the skin, joints of the head, face, and neck including hearing, balance, and taste are all under the control of the brainstem. Control of the trunk and limbs for both sensation and motor control is mediated by the spinal cord (Kelly & Dodd, 2000).

The medulla actually is an enlargement of the top of the spinal cord and occasionally is referred to as the bulb. This structure is extremely important for speech motor control. It contains both ascending and descending nerve tracts as well as the nuclei of the cranial nerves controlling phonation, articula-

tion, velopharyngeal closure, and swallowing. The medulla contains cells of the reticular activating formation that is crucial for overall arousal and important for sleep.

The pons is located superiorly to the medulla and inferior to the midbrain. It contains the nuclei for the trigeminal, abducens, facial, and vestibulocochlear nerves. It is the "bridge" to the cerebellum. The pons also helps control breathing and sleep and contains part of the reticular activating system, which is important for alertness and arousal functioning.

The midbrain contains most of the brainstem and connects it to the forebrain. It contains the superior colliculus for vision and inferior colliculus for hearing. It also houses the nuclei for the oculomotor and trochlear cranial nerves, important for eye movement and sensation. The substantia nigra is also housed in the midbrain. The substantia nigra produces the neurotransmitter dopamine and plays an important role in the reward center. It is responsible for controlling sensory processes such as vision and movement. A common disorder affecting this region (specifically the substantia nigra) is Parkinson's disease.

The 12 Cranial Nerves

There are 12 pairs of cranial nerves. With the exception of cranial nerve I (olfactory) and II (optic), the cranial nerves emanate from the brainstem. They serve functions that are motor (efferent), sensory (afferent), or both. Motor nerves send impulses from the cortex via neural pathways to the spinal cord. Once there, they synapse with the cell bodies in the spinal cord. The nerve impulses are then sent to the targeted muscles, glands, or organs via the peripheral nervous system. The motor nerves include the occulomotor (III), trochlear, (IV), abducens (VI), spinal accessory (XI), and the hypoglossal (XII). Sensory nerves receive input from the periphery and send nerve impulses from the sensory organs to the brain. The sensory portions of the cranial nerves have their origin outside the brain in ganglia that divide into two branches: one that extends into the post-central gyrus (the sensory cortex) and one that connects to the sensory organ itself. The sensory nerves include the olfactory (I), optic (II), and the vestibulocochlear (VIII). Mixed nerves have more

Table 1–2. Cranial Nerves

I. Olfactory (smell)

II. Optic (vision)

III. Oculomotor (eye movement and pupil constriction)

IV. Trochlear (eye movement)

V. Trigeminal (sensations of touch, pain, and temperature from the face and head; chewing and swallowing)

VI. Abducens (eye movement)

VII. Facial (taste for anterior 2/3 of tongue, somatosensory information from ear, facial expression, controls muscles for facial expression)

VIII. Acoustic/Vestibulocochlear (hearing and balance)

IX. Glossopharyngeal (taste for posterior half of tongue and somatosensory information from tongue, tonsils, and pharynx, and controls some muscles for swallowing)

X. Vagus (sensory, motor, and autonomic visceral functions: heart rate, glands, digestion)

XI. (Spinal) Accessory (controls muscles used in head movement)

XII. Hypoglossal (controls muscles of tongue)

The following Web site provides an overview of the cranial nerves with their associated locations: http://faculty.washington.edu/chudler/cranial .html

than one originating nucleus and include the trigeminal nerve (V), the facial nerve (VII), the glossopharygeal (IX) and the vagus nerve (X) (Table 1–2).

Subcortical Structures

Subcortical structures are found above the midbrain and contain the hypothalamus and thalamus, also referred to as the diencephalon. The thalamus is an oval structure that acts as the gatekeeper to relay sensory input to other areas of the brain. It is located in the center of the forebrain. Most sensory information is processed first in the thalamus and then is relayed to the cerebral cortex. Thalamic lesions may affect contralateral somatic sensations and create a lower threshold for pain. The hypothalamus is a small area located ventral to the thalamus with widespread connections to the thalamus, reticular formation, cerebral cortex, limbic system, olfactory bulb, and midbrain. Its many nuclei help regulate endocrine functions. Damage to one of the hypothalamic nuclei often leads to difficulty with feeding, drinking, temperature regulation, sexual behavior, sleep, wakefulness, activity level, and/or fighting. The hypothalamus also exerts a major influence on regulating the body's hormonal system and can impact emotional expression, food intake, metabolism, and cycles of sleep and wakefulness as well. Attached to the base of the hypothalamus is the pituitary gland. It releases hormones into the bloodstream and to other organs. It is considered the master gland of the body controlling secretions from the thyroid, adrenal gland, ovaries, and testes.

The hippocampus is another subcortical structure located between the thalamus and cerebral cortex and is important for recent working memory. It is also crucial for inhibiting a habitually unsuccessful action. The amygdala also plays a role in memory. The amygdala's primary role is in forming

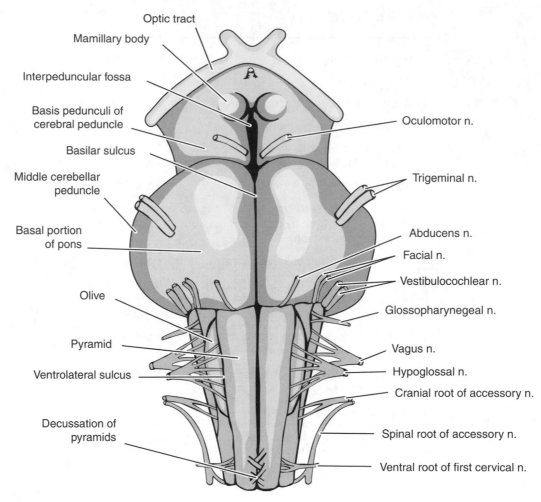

Optic tract
Mamillary body
Interpeduncular fossa
Basis pedunculi of cerebral peduncle
Basilar sulcus
Middle cerebellar peduncle
Basal portion of pons
Olive
Pyramid
Ventrolateral sulcus
Decussation of pyramids

Oculomotor n.
Trigeminal n.
Abducens n.
Facial n.
Vestibulocochlear n.
Glossopharynegeal n.
Vagus n.
Hypoglossal n.
Cranial root of accessory n.
Spinal root of accessory n.
Ventral root of first cervical n.

Figure 1–9. Brainstem.

and storing memories associated with emotional events. The hippocampus and the amygdala work as a whole system to regulate motivation and emotions (Figure 1-10).

The Cerebellum

The cerebellum is inferior to the occipital lobes and posterior to the brainstem. The cerebellum has two hemispheres and is divided into three lobes each. The white matter within the cerebellum connects it to other parts of the central nervous system. The gray matter analyzes body movement and compares it to what is needed to accomplish a specific motor task. It is crucial for maintaining balance in space and executing coordinated movements. A very critical function of this structure for speech and swallowing is the integration of sensory input from regions of the brain, allowing it to coordinate muscle groups. The cerebellum also modifies muscle tone, speed, and range of motion, allowing movements to be executed smoothly.

The cerebellum helps to make sequenced motor skills automatic. Since the cerebellum is important for motor control, it receives input from muscle spindles and tendons via the spinal cord. It also gets input from vision, hearing, touch, and the vestibular

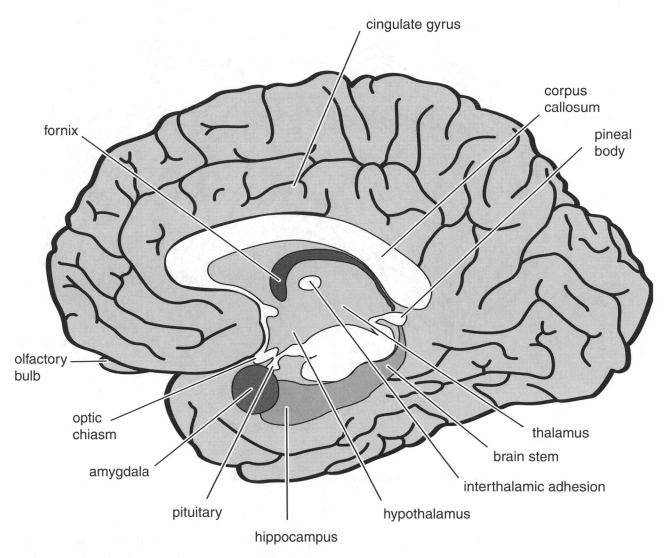

Figure 1–10. Subcortical structures of brain.

system for balance. A critical distinction between the cerebellum and the cortical structures is that the cerebellum can only control and perform online correction of planned movements. It does not initiate motor activity (Figure 1-11).

Neural Pathways

To the left and right of the thalamus is the basal ganglia, which includes the caudate nucleus, putamen, and globus pallidus. These structures are involved in motor control and integration. They form part of the extrapyramidal system, which are neural pathways whose function is the coordination of involuntary movement. The anatomy of the extrapyramidal system remains unclear. It primarily connects the cortex with the basal ganglia but it also has indirect influence on the the lower motor neuron in the spinal cord. This system is polysynaptic, that is, it makes many connections through interneurons before its impulses reach the spinal cord. These tracts affect

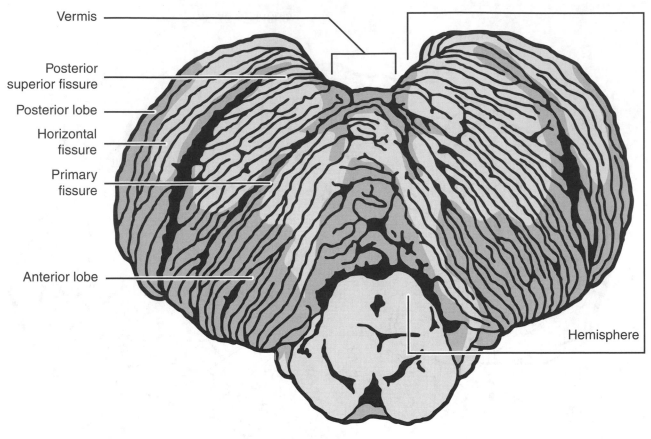

Vermis

Posterior
superior fissure

Posterior lobe

Horizontal
fissure

Primary
fissure

Anterior lobe

Hemisphere

Figure 1–11. Cerebellum.

reflexes, locomotion, posture, and complex movement. Any degradation of the extrapyramidal system due to stroke or other neurological processes causes difficulties with motor control. People with extrapyramidal disorders have varied clinical presentations. They may have difficulty initiating movement (akinesia) or inability to remain still or motionless (akathisia). Tardive dyskinesia, commonly seen as a side effect from prolonged use of some psychotropic drugs is manifested as involuntary and irregular muscle movement. Cerebral palsy of the athetoid type is another example of an extrapyramidal disorder. Huntington's chorea and Parkinson's disease are the best known examples of extrapyramidal disorders and many speech-language pathologists who practice in an acute-care setting will encounter these patients. The extrapyramidal system plays a significant role in speech production and swallowing

function and every speech and language clinician must be aware of its structure and functions.

The pyramidal system consists of upper motor neurons in the primary motor cortex whose axons synapse with the lower motor neurons in the anterior horn of the spinal cord. The lower motor neuron axon, also referred to as the final common pathway or the alpha-neuron, begins in the spinal cord and extends to the muscles for movement of the arms and legs. The pyramidal system is a monosynatpic system and controls all voluntary movement. It is made up of three nerve tracts: the corticospinal, the corticobulbar, and the corticopontine. The corticospinal tract controls the movements of the limbs and digits. Eighty to ninety percent of corticospinal tract axons cross over to the other side in the medulla. This crossover is referred to as the point of pryamidal decussation. Injuries to upper motor neurons in the cortex at the point before they enter the pyramidal decussation will lead to spastic paralysis on the opposite side of the body. If an injury occurs to the pyramidal tract below the point of decussation, or to the lower motor neurons in the spinal cord, paralysis on the same side of the body will result. The axons of the corticobulbar tract synapse with the cranial nerves and therefore affect the movement of the speech musculature. The corticopontine tract connects the nuclei in the pons to the cerebellum. After receiving information from sensory input, it is the pyramidal system that activates muscles so that various body parts can move as needed (Figure 1–12).

Cerebral Blood Flow

The brain is only 2% of the average adult body weight. However, it receives 15% of the total cardiac output, and uses 25% of the total body glucose. It also consumes almost 20% of available oxygen within the entire body.

There are two broad arterial systems: the carotid and the vertebrobasilar (Figure 1–13). The carotid arterial system has a left and right branch and divides into the internal and external carotid arteries. The internal carotids supply the blood to the anterior part of the brain and subdivide into the anterior cerebral artery (ACA), middle cerebral artery (MCA), and the posterior cerebral artery (PCA). The external carotid artery supplies blood to the face, the tongue, and parts of the head.

The Circle of Willis is a critical structure because it allows blood to flow through both hemispheres of the brain and acts as a safety valve if blood flow on one side of the brain is blocked. Due to its construction, if blood flow is blocked on the left, blood from the right can reach the unnourished area (Love & Webb, 1992). Branching off from the Circle of Willis are two arterial systems that supply the forebrain and cortical areas pertinent to speech and language production: the anterior communicating artery (ACA) and the middle cerebral artery (MCA). The posterior cortex, the midbrain, and the brainstem are all supplied by the posterior cerebral artery, the basilar artery, and the vertebral artery.

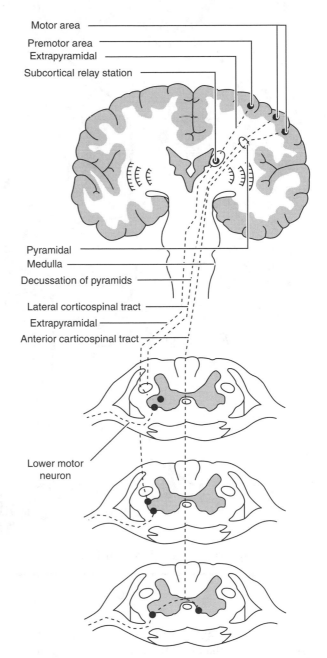

Figure 1–12. Extrapyramidal and pyramidal systems.

The anterior cerebral artery supplies blood to the medial surfaces of the frontal and parietal cortex. The middle cerebral artery supplies most of the lateral cortex of both cerebral hemispheres, including portions of the temporal lobes and frontal lobes. It provides blood flow to both Broca's and Wernicke's

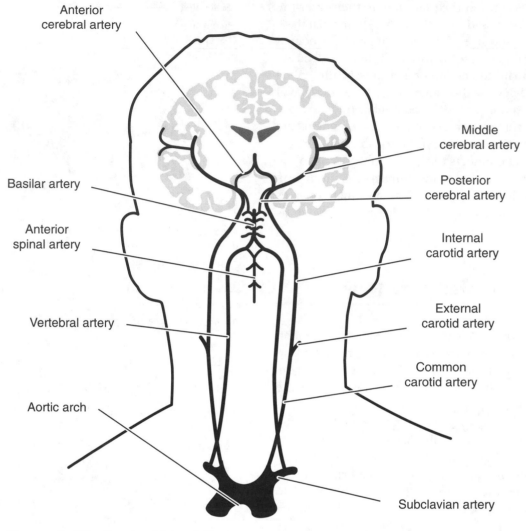

Anterior
cerebral artery

Basilar artery

Anterior
spinal artery

Vertebral artery

Aortic arch

Middle
cerebral artery

Posterior
cerebral artery

Internal
carotid artery

External
carotid artery

Common
carotid artery

Subclavian artery

Figure 1–13. Cerebral blood flow.

areas. It also has smaller branches that supply blood to the basal ganglia and internal capsule. The posterior cerebral history supplies medial and inferior surfaces of occipital and temporal lobes. The vertebrobasilar arterial system supplies the occipital lobes, medial aspects of the temporal lobes and brainstem.

Cerebrovascular Accidents

Cerebrovascular accident (CVA), commonly known as stroke, refers to a lack of blood flow to any area of the brain, including the brainstem. As the brain is

not able to store oxygen or glucose, any interruption of blood flow affects its ability to function properly. The cerebral arteries supply oxygen and blood to parts of the brain. The cerebral arteries arise from the internal carotid and vertebral arteries. At the base of the brain the arteries form the Circle of Willis. It is there that branches of the internal carotid arteries and branches of the basilar arteries communicate. The middle cerebral artery (MCA) is the largest of the cerebral arteries (compared to the anterior cerebral artery and the posterior cerebral artery). The MCA is most often related to a CVA as it supplies blood and oxygen to most of the outer surface of the brain, the basal ganglia, and anterior and posterior internal capsules (Slater, 2006). Cerebral infarcts which disrupt blood flow and oxygen to the brain may arise from hemorrhagic or ischemic events in any of the arteries.

In the United States, there are 700,000 strokes annually. It is the third leading cause of death in the country and the leading cause of long-term disability (National Institute of Neurological Disorders and Stroke, 2008). Both the ischemic and hemorrhagic types of stroke are considered cerebral vascular accidents and can cause aphasia. There are approximately 100,000 cases of aphasia annually in the United States due to stroke alone (Helm-Estabrooks & Albert, 2004).

Hemorrhagic Events

The hemorrhagic stroke typifies approximately 20% of all strokes. However, the mortality rate of hemorrhagic strokes is 50% in the United States. These strokes can be due to massive edema, brain herniation, or the use of illicit drugs, especially cocaine. Other etiologies include aneurysm, clotting deficiencies, leukemia, brain tumors, and occasionally traumatic brain injury. A majority of hemorrhagic strokes are due to the rupture of a congenital berry aneurysm. In the United States, approximately one-fourth of people who suffer a stroke will die. About one-half will live with long-term disabilities, and another one-fourth will recover mostly all functions (National Institutes of Health, 2008) (Figure 1–14A).

Ischemic Events

There are two types of ischemic stroke, thrombotic and embolic. The thrombotic type is due to a blood clot that forms in a vessel and remains there. Fat and blood from the diseased artery block the vessel going to the brain and the artery narrows at the site of the thrombosis. The embolic type is caused by a blood clot that travels from the site where it was formed to a cerebral artery. The detached mass within the blood vessel is carried along with the blood flow, preventing nutrients such as oxygen and glucose from nourishing the cortical tissue. Approximately 80% of all strokes are of this type (NINDS, 2008). Lacunar infarcts are a type of ischemic stroke. This results from constriction of the small vessels that penetrate the brain, usually caused by hypertension. Finally, lacunar disease also can be caused by transient ischemic attacks (TIA), which are brief events, lasting less than 24 hours. They typically last only two to 15 minutes without evidence of brain damage (Figure 1–14B).

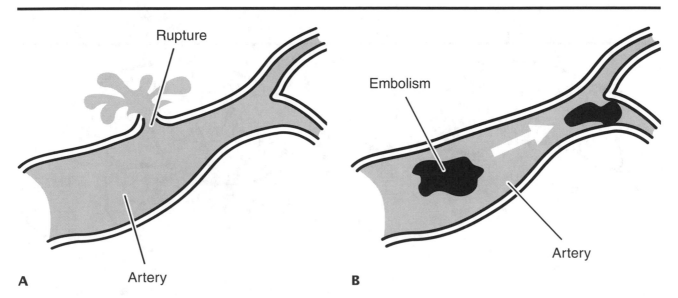

Figure 1–14. (**A**) Hemorrhagic event, and (**B**) ischemic event.

Potential Sequelae to Anterior Cerebral Artery (ACA) Stroke

From the internal carotid artery, the anterior cerebral artery extends both forward and upward. It supplies blood to the frontal lobes. This part of the brain impacts personality, logical thought, and voluntary movement, particularly in the legs. Damage to this area due to stroke may result in weakness of the opposite leg; however, damage to both anterior cerebral territories may produce an akinetic form of mutism (DeFelice, 2005; Stroke Center at Washington University, 2008).

Damage to the ACA (Figure 1–15) may result in:

- Confusion
- Loss of coordination
- Impaired sensory functions
- Personality changes
- Contralateral paresis or paralysis

Potential Sequelae to Middle Cerebral Artery (MCA) Stroke

The middle cerebral artery provides blood to much of the temporal lobe, anterolateral frontal lobe, and parietal lobe. Damage to this area may result in a homonymous hemianopsia which is commonly expressed in ipsilateral head or eye deviation. Contralateral hemiplegia concerning the face, arm, and to a less significant extent, the leg, is also noted. Typically, the blockage is embolic although thrombotic blockage is frequently seen in the carotid (DeFelice, 2005; Slater, 2006).

Damage to the MCA (Figure 1–16) may result in:

- Aphasic syndromes
- Motor speech disorders
- Visual field cuts
- Contralateral paresis or paralysis

Potential Sequelae to Posterior Cerebral Artery (PCA) Stroke

The posterior cerebral artery provides blood to the occipital lobe and the inferior section of the temporal lobe, originating from the basilar artery. When this area is damaged, problems with vision, memory, smell, and emotion may arise in conjunction with functions associated with the midbrain and thalamus (DeFelice, 2005)

Damage to the PCA (Figure 1–17) may result in:

- Visual field cut
- Sensory impairment
- Alexia
- Cortical blindness
- Color blindness
- Locked-in syndrome
- Agnosias

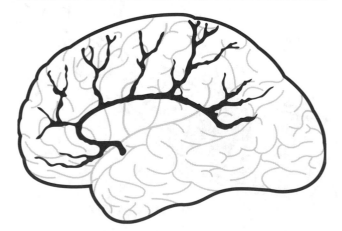

Figure 1–15. Anterior cerebral arteries.

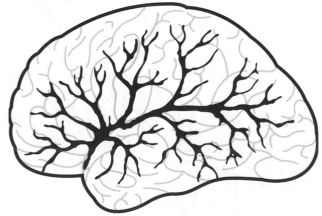

Figure 1–16. Middle cerebral arteries.

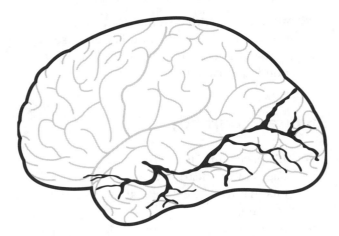

Figure 1–17. Posterior cerebral arteries.

Brain Imaging and Selected Medical Tests for Acquired Language Disorders

The medical diagnosis of stroke includes imaging studies, that is, tests that provide static or dynamic images of the damaged areas of the brain to supplement the clinical findings. Some of these tests image blood flow and metabolic activity, and some image structure. Some use radioactive materials and some do not. The most frequently used imaging studies used in the diagnosis of stroke include: CT scan, MRI, and SPECT scan. In addition to imaging studies, the major cerebral arteries and blood flow may be tested via Doppler ultrasound, carotid phonoangiography, encardiography, or angiography. Several brain imaging tests are outlined below.

CAT Scan or CT Scan (Computerized Axial Tomography)

- This test takes 10 to 20 minutes to conduct.
- A 3-D picture is created from different angles in slices, linked to x-rays to detect hemorrhages, lesions, and tumors.
- Must be done to detect if a stroke is hemorrhagic or ischemic (important to know prior to giving tPA—tissue plasminogen activator).
- This is not a good test for soft tissue lesions.
- This is a good test for pinpointing site of lesion.

MRI—Magnetic Resonance Imaging

- Testing time is typically 30 to 45 minutes.
- A magnetic field is used to show fine details in the brain and spinal cord.
- MRI shows:
  - soft tissues
  - large blood vessels
  - location and size of arteriovenous malformations
  - tumors
  - blood clots
  - ischemic stroke

fMRI—Functional Magnetic Resonance Imaging

- fMRI is a nonradioactive, noninvasive procedure that shows the use of glucose and oxygen feeding areas of the working brain.
- Movement of the patient during the procedure can adversely affect readings.
- fMRI can be used:
  - to map critical areas in patients prior to brain surgery
  - to identify CNS and some psychiatric disorders
  - to measure therapeutic effects of neurologic disorders

PET Scan (Positron Emission Tomography)

This test is radioactive and provides imaging of metabolic activity in the brain:

- The radioactive markers assess the brain's metabolism for oxygen and glucose and blood flow.
- This test reveals how the brain is using blood flow to function.
- This test is expensive and not done routinely as a diagnostic tool but more often for research purposes in clinical settings.

SPECT Scan (Single Photon Emission Computerized Tomography)

- This test evaluates the amount of blood flowing through the brain's regions.
- It can identify areas of reduced or absent blood flow (known as regional cerebral blood flow or rCBF).
- This test assesses cerebral metabolism of glucose and oxygen.
- It typically is not done as an inpatient procedure due to its high expense.
- SPECT is more commonly used for research purposes.

Examination of the Carotids: Doppler Ultrasound or Auscultation of the Carotids

- Doppler examination of the carotids use an ultrasound technique with high-frequency sound waves.
- This is a noninvasive procedure that examines the blood flow in the major arteries and veins of the neck and brain.
- This examination detects bruits which are turbulent sounds within an artery and indicate extracranial carotid occlusive disease.
- Audio measurements "hear" the blood flow and produce a visual image of the carotid arteries.
- This procedure is used in patients with vascular disease to identify partial or complete occlusion of a vessel.

- Auscultation with a stethoscope also provides evidence of carotid artery disease through the detection of the turbulent sounds associated with bruits.

Endocardiography

- This procedure uses ultrasound to take images of the heart and can detect blood clots that have the potential to travel to the brain.
- Endocardiography can detect:
  - a hole in the atrium of the heart
  - a clot in a ventricle
  - an infected valve of the heart
  - an enlarged heart that is a risk factor for stroke (often due to chronic hypertension)

Angiography

- CT Type (Computed Tomography)
  - A trace element is injected intravenously with contrast dye to detect blood flow.
  - Ischemic areas or a subaracnoid aneurysm can be detected.
  - This test delineates areas where there is a deprivation of blood flow.
- MR Type (Magnetic Resonance)
  - This test is similar to an MRI but is conducted with contrast dye that is injected to depict blood flow to the brain.
- Cerebral Angiography
  - This is an invasive test using dye that is injected intravenously into an artery.
  - A catheter is surgically inserted into a blood vessel around the groin which is guided through the circulatory system to an artery leading to the brain.
  - X-rays are taken to track blood flow.
  - Abnormalities that can cause stroke (aneurysm, narrowing vessels, embolus, atherosclerosis, arteriovenous malformations, etc.) can be detected.

■ There is a risk to this procedure. If a clot is present in the artery prior to the procedure, introducing the catheter into the artery can dislodge the clot, thereby increasing the probability of an embolic stroke.

References

Bhatnagar, S. C. (2002). Nerve cells. *Neuroscience for the study of communicative disorders* (2nd ed.). Philadelphia: Lippincott Williams & Wilkins.

DeFelice, E. A. (2005). *Prevention of cardiovascular disease: Atherosclerosis, carotid artery disease, cerebral artery disease/stroke, coronary artery disease, peripheral artery disease and hypertension.* Lincoln, NE: iUniverse.

Helm-Estabrooks, N., & Albert, M. L. (2004). *Manual of aphasia and aphasia therapy* (2nd ed.). Austin, TX: Pro-Ed.

Kelly, J. P., & Dodd, J. (2000). Anatomical organization of the nervous system. In E. R. Kandel, J. H. Schwartz, & T. M. Jessell (Eds.), *Principles of neural science* (4th ed.). Columbus, OH: McGraw-Hill.

National Institutes of Health. (2008). *Medline plus outlook on stroke.* Retrieved July 26, 2008, from http://www.nlm.nih.gov/medlineplus/ency/article/000761.htm#Expectations%20(prognosis)

National Institute of Neurological Disorders and Stroke. (2008). *What you need to know about stroke.* Retrieved July 26, 2008, from http://www.ninds.nih.gov/disorders/stroke/stroke_needtoknow.htm

Schwartz, J. H. (1991). Chemical messengers: Small molecules and peptides. In E. R. Kandel, J. H. Schwartz, & T. M. Jessell (Eds.), *Principles of neural science* (4th ed.). Norwalk, CT: Appleton and Lange.

Slater, D. I. (2006). *Middle cerebral artery stroke.* Retrieved July 26, 2008, from http://www.emedicine.com/pmr/TOPIC77.HTM

Stroke Center at Washington University. (2008). *Blood vessels of the brain.* Retrieved July 26, 2008, from http://www.strokecenter.org/education/ais_vessels/ais049a.html

Webb, W., & Adler, R. K. (2008). *Neurology for the speech-language pathologist* (5th ed.). St. Louis, MO: Mosby-Elsevier.

Chapter 2

ASSESSMENT AND TREATMENT PROCESSES IN ACQUIRED LANGUAGE DISORDERS

Assessment

The purpose of the initial evaluation is to determine if the person has aphasia, to classify the type of aphasia, its level of severity, and to provide a functional prognosis. Throughout the therapeutic course functional communication is emphasized and the SLP gauges the patient's recovery by charting changes in the areas of impairment. The speech-language pathologist (SLP) obtains important information about the patient and family during the initial interview process, which informs the development of a functional and meaningful treatment plan. A case history is obtained from the medical chart or during the interview and typically includes the following information:

- Chief complaints and admitting diagnosis
- Past medical history (PMH)
- Past surgical history
- Family history
- Psychosocial history
- Work and educational history

If the clinician sees the patient in an inpatient setting, it is always best practice to contact family members/caregivers to confirm the information that the patient provided as well as to obtain another perspective on the patient and his or her history. Information about the patient's communica-

tion style and communicative needs in the home environment should be obtained. It is said that the eyes and ears of a clinician are sometimes the best diagnostic tools available. Consequently, informal observational findings supplement and complement the formal diagnostic testing. Using both informal and formal methods of assessment further help the SLP in the development of a proper plan of treatment. Areas of speech and language to evaluate are:

- Discourse ability (conversations and questions)
- Auditory comprehension (following commands)
- Naming skills (clothing, accessories, money, etc.)
- Repetition skills (words, sentences with increasing syllables)
- Reading and writing (read printed words and write names of objects)
- Ability to sing ("Happy Birthday")
- Praxis (waving, hammering, blowing out candles, etc.)

In addition to the case history and speech-language findings, the clinician needs to be alert to the following information and integrate it into her clinical picture of the patient. This information can be obtained from the medical chart, specifically in the nursing notes and the consults from other services in the hospital who are also involved in the patient's care.

- Behavior
- Gait and posture
- Appearance
- Gross functioning of skin, head, neck, and spine
- Noted impairment in cranial nerves
- Reflexes
- Stereognosis (identify object felt in hand without visual help)

Aspects of the motor system should also be noted:

- Muscle tone and strength
- Muscle wasting
- Physical symmetry
- Coordination (balance, walking, sitting)
- Involuntary movements (shaking, twitching, tremors)

See the Speech-Language Pathology Case History Form provided (Appendix A).

Areas of Language Function

Six major areas of language functioning are generally considered when assessing aphasia. These areas are noted below as well as the most common lesion sites producing the aphasic symptoms

1. The first area is the patient's **speech fluency**. Fluency involves the length of the utterance that an individual expresses in connected words. Fluent speech generally includes phrases and sentences that are at least 4 words in length. Fluent aphasias involve a more posterior lesion (around the temporoparietal junction) in the cerebral cortex whereas non-fluent aphasias generally result from a more anterior lesion (the perisylvian gyrus) in the brain.
2. The second area of assessment involves **comprehension of language**. Patients with more posterior lesions typically have more comprehen-sion difficulties than those with anterior lesions. Comprehension is a broad term and can involve understanding words, phrases, sentences, para-graphs, stories, and conversation.
3. The third area of assessment involves the ability to use **automatic speech**. Automatic speech refers to commonly used sequences of language. For example, days of the week and months of the year are considered automatic. This type of language tends to be easier to produce as it becomes rote over time.
4. The fourth area of assessment is **repetition or imitative speech**. The ability to repeat what one hears is a diagnostic feature. Individuals with certain types of aphasia (such as conduc-tion aphasia) have difficulty with repetition of speech.
5. The fifth area of assessment is **naming**. Struggle, circumlocutions, recurrent utterances, parapha-sias, jargon, and confrontation naming difficulty can be observed in patients with naming problems.
6. The sixth area of assessment is **grammatical use**. Agrammatism, which is typical for anterior lesions, is characterized by fragmented, incom-plete use of sentences and includes omissions and substitutions of inflections and function words (prepositions, articles, conjunctions, etc.). Speech may sound telegraphic. Agrammatism is often prevalent in those with a nonfluent type of aphasia. Paragrammatism indicates a reduced syntactic complexity with substitution of func-tion words and inflections. This tends to coin-cide with paraphasic errors often seen in fluent types of aphasia and is more consistent with a posterior lesion. Table 2–1 provides an over-view of the characteristics of the major aphasic syndromes.

Characteristics of Major Aphasic Syndromes

Each of the major aphasic syndromes have both shared and unique characteristics. In reality, very few of them are "pure" and people with aphasia often have overlapping features. The categories listed below

Table 2–1. Characteristics of the Major Aphasic Syndromes

	Paragraph Comprehension	Automatic Speech	Verbal Repetition	Word Recall	Grammar	Fluency
Broca's Aphasia	Good	Good	Fair	Latencies struggle	Agrammatic	Nonfluent
Wernicke's Aphasia	Poor	Poor	Poor	Circumlocutions	Paragrammatic	Fluent Paraphasic
Conduction Aphasia	Good	Varies	Poor	Varies	Varies	Fluent Paraphasic
Global Aphasia	Poor	Poor	Poor	Nonverbal or recurrent utterances	Agrammatic	Nonfluent except for recurrent utterances
Transcortical Sensory Aphasia	Poor	Poor	Excellent	Paraphasia Jargon	Paragrammatic	Fluent Paraphasic
Transcortical Motor Aphasia	Good	Good	Excellent	Good Confrontation	Varies	Combined
Anomic Aphasia	Good	Good	Good	Latencies and/or circumlocutions	Good	Fluent

are the primary characteristics used to assist in the differential diagnosis of the syndromes (Figure 2–1). In our discussion of the major aphasic syndromes, we assume that the left hemisphere is dominant for speech and language functions.

Just as the aphasic syndromes commonly seen in the clinical setting have both shared and unique characteristics, each syndrome can have more than one name. For example, Broca's aphasia is also known as an *anterior aphasia, motor aphasia, nonfluent aphasia,* and sometimes, *expressive aphasia.* Wernicke's aphasia is sometimes referred to as a *posterior aphasia, fluent aphasia, sensory aphasia,* or *receptive aphasia.* The interchangeability of these terms reflects the culture of the medical setting and not a nosological difference.

The major aphasic syndromes noted above are due to cortical lesions. However, it is also possible to see aphasia secondary to a subcortical lesion. There are two major types of subcortical aphasia. One is due to a lesion in the basal ganglia and adja-

cent regions of the internal capsule. The other is due to a lesion in the left thalamus. These are discussed in detail in the chapter on subcortical aphasia (Chapter 5).

Definitions of the Clinical Characteristics of the Major Aphasic Syndromes

Fluency. Fluency refers to the ability to produce an uninterrupted, phrase-length utterance, typically more than 4 words in length.

Prosody. Prosody involves the ability to vary intonation patterns, stress, and rhythm in connected speech.

Auditory Comprehension. Auditory comprehension involves the ability to listen to and process information presented verbally. This ranges in levels from the ability to comprehend at the word level to the conversational level.

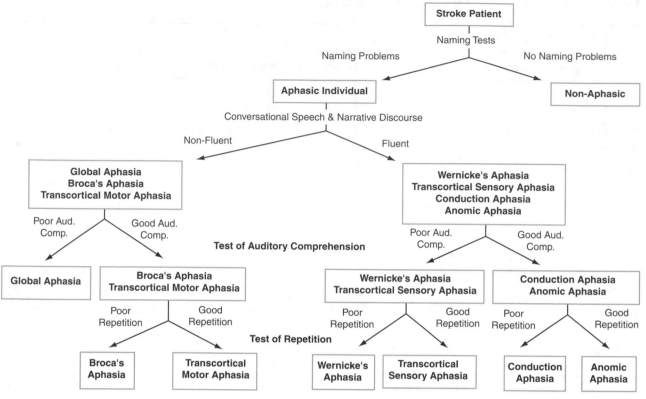

Figure 2–1. Characteristics of major aphasic syndromes.

From Helm-Estabrooks, N. & Albert, M. (1991). *Manual of aphasia therapy*. Austin, TX: Pro-Ed. Reprinted with permission.

Automatic Speech. Automatic speech involves the ability to produce rote sequences such as counting, naming the days of the week, the months of the year, and so forth.

Verbal Repetition. Verbal repetition requires the ability to repeat what the examiner said. This skill is initially assessed from the monosyllabic level to sentence imitation.

Word Recall. Word recall refers to the ability to name objects and pictures during structured confrontation naming as well as at the conversational level. This can also be referred to as *lexical retrieval, or word finding.*

Syntax. Syntactic ability involves organization of words and sentences into a logical structures based on the rules of syntax for a particular language. **Agrammatism** occurs in individuals with nonfluent aphasia and is characterized by the absence of functor words, thereby creating sentences that include primarily nouns and verbs. The speech is telegraphic and there can be omissions of grammatical morphemes. **Paragrammatism** occurs in fluent aphasia and is characterized by inaccurate syntactic rule application, for example, subject-verb agreement or incorrect tense markers, and inappropriate use of pronouns.

Perseveration. Perseveration is defined as the *inappropriate repetition of a previous response that continues after the task requirements have changed and the response is no longer needed.* There are three primary types of perseveration: *stuck-in-set, continuous,* and *recurrent.* Table 2–2 provides a definition and an example of each of these types of perseveration.

Ideational perseveration also may be observed in some patients. In this type, the patient persev-

Table 2–2. Primary Types of Perseveration

Type	Definition	Example
Stuck-in-set Perseveration *Lesion:* More frontal	Inappropriate maintenance of a category or framework after a new task is introduced and a new response expected	Working on naming within a food category. When the task is changed to clothing, the patient continues to assign food names to the items of clothing.
Continuous Perseveration *Lesion:* Right hemispheric, subcortical and cortical aphasias	Inappropriate prolongation of a behavior that should stop; inability to inhibit the continuation of the response	Erasing an incorrect response as directed, but continuing until the paper is torn.
Recurrent Perseveration *Lesion:* Left temporal and parietal region	Inappropriate recurrence of a previous response after a new stimulus is given and a new response expected	There can be a carryover of whole words (perseverates on *slipper* for all stimuli in the semantic category of "footwear"); or carryover of phonemic structure (perseverates on /k/ in initial position for all words subsequent to the first presentation of /k/)

erates on a concept or idea despite a topic shift or change in communicative context. For example, continuing to talk about the breakfast meal, even though the topic has switched to daily activities that occur after eating breakfast. Studies indicate that 63 to 87% of aphasics have some degree of perseveration. Many people with aphasia have recurrent perseveration. There appears to be no difference in the rates of perseveration between fluent and nonfluent patients with aphasia (Helm-Estabrooks & Albert, 2004).

One must also be attentive during diagnostic testing because some errors that appear perseverative may actually be showing the therapist that the patient may have understood the task. For example, the patient may point to his head then his toe in response to your directive to point to the ceiling then the floor. However, earlier, you were asking him to point to body parts. In this case, the patient understood the directionality of the directive, but perseverated on body parts.

Clinical observations of patients with perseverative behavior have shown that certain tasks or contexts will increase the likelihood of its occurrence. This is a very important fact for a treating therapist to understand since the reduction and/or elimination of perseveration is a crucial factor for successful functional communication.

The following tasks are likely to increase the likelihood of perseveration:

- Tasks that involve nonautomatic speech will increase perseveration. For example, naming tasks will increase perseveration versus counting to 10 or reciting the days of the week.
- Tasks that involve naming items, pictures, or objects that are in similar semantic fields will increase perseveration. For example, having a patient name fruits and then switch the task to naming vegetables will increase the likelihood that they will continue to name fruits (recurrent perseveration).
- Tasks that require the patient to respond more rapidly between trials will increase perseveration.
- Tasks that require the use of lexical items that occur less frequently in the language will increase perseveration. For example, this may include asking the patient to name geometric shapes such as hexagon, rectangle, and octagon.
- Tasks that use words that are close in semantic and/or phonemic properties can cause increased perseveration. For example, requiring a patient to name the following

pictures: *dog, doctor, door, cat, nurse, window* may present a challenge. The semantic proximity of the words *doctor* and *nurse*, and *cat* and *dog*; the phonemic proximity of the words, *door, doctor, dog* can also increase perseveration. Consequently, the word *window* may not be produced successfully.

It is possible to decrease perseveration although it can be quite intractable. Helms-Estabrooks (1987) developed the Treatment of Aphasic Perseveration (TAP) program. In this program, the therapist writes the word that the patient is repeating on a piece of paper. One technique is to cross out the word in an attempt to extinguish the perseveration, while the patient watches. The therapist tells that patient that she no longer needs to say this word. Other techniques to control or reduce perseveration include:

- Establish new rules for new tasks: "Now we are going to stop talking about animals. We will now talk about clothing."
- Give the patient a break by using a distracting comment: "Do you think it will rain today?"
- Raise the patient's level of awareness about his perseveration: "You are repeating the same word over again, John. Do you hear yourself?"
- Do not allow the patient to see any written work that he has done earlier in the session, which can be a perseverative stimulus.

Paraphasia. Aphasic speech can be characterized by paraphasic errors, although not all patients dem-

onstrate this particular characteristic. These errors reflect a disruption at the lexical level, for semantic paraphasias, or the phonological level, for the phonemic paraphasias. For more information see Kohn (1989, 1993) and Caplan (1987). There are three general types of paraphasias: phonemic, semantic, and neologistic (often referred to as a *neologism*). A *phonemic paraphasia* is characterized by a similar word substitution, where at least 50% of the word overlaps phonologically with the intended word. Examples include saying "octagon" for "octopus," or "ship" for "shirt." Phonemic paraphasias may also take the phonological shape of a nonword, for example, "ocoput" for "octopus." This is referred to as a *non-word phonemic paraphasia*. A *semantic paraphasia* is a verbal paraphasia related to the target word, for example, "jellyfish" for "octopus." This is referred to as a *related semantic paraphasia* because it is in the same class as the intended word. The *unrelated semantic paraphasia* is a real word, but not in the same class, for example, "chicken" for "octopus." Semantic paraphasias are also known as *verbal paraphasias*. A neologism is not a real word phonologically or semantically, for example, the neologism "ertig" may be said for "octopus." Notice, however, that the neologism follows the phonological rules of English, yet it is not a real word. Figure 2–2 maps the relationships of the three primary types of paraphasias.

Error Recognition. This involves the ability to recognize a phonemic (literal), semantic (verbal) or neologistic self-generated error. For individuals with error recognition problems, they are not aware that their speech contains the wrong sound, the wrong word or a nonword.

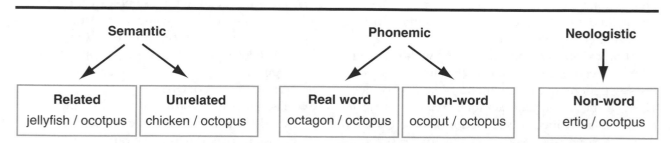

Figure 2–2. A mapping of the relationships of the three primary types of paraphasias.

Types of Assessment

Functional Assessment

Functional testing is important to helping patients function most successfully in the world. A breakdown of visually mediated and verbally mediated functions of receptive and expressive language is delineated in Figure 2–3. There are many measures such as *Focus on Function* (2nd edition, Klein & Hahn, 2007) that provide numerous functional activities for patients in therapy. Primary areas include:

- Basic Communication, including expressing ideas and starting conversations
- Using the Phone, including making appointments and taking messages
- Managing and Understanding Time, including designing a schedule and using a calendar
- Managing and Understanding Finances, including check writing and using an ATM
- Shopping, including working with money and using coupons
- Meals and Cooking, including planning menus, writing shopping lists, and cooking
- Getting Around, including reading and understanding signs, symbols and maps
- Activities around the House, including ordering, reading directions, writing letters
- Social Participation, including social exchanges and discussing feelings and emotions
- Leisure Activities, including using the internet and communicating via E-mail
- Work-Related Tasks, including resume writing and completing applications

Appendix B (Skills Assessment Inventory) provides a checklist of functional topics that adults typically engage in during activities of daily living (ADLs).

The American Speech-Language-Hearing Association Functional Assessment of Communication Skills for Adults (ASHA FACS) (1995) is designed for assessing functional skills of adults in the rehabilitative process. The ASHA FACS provides a conceptual framework and measurement tool to assess four domains: (1) social communication, (2) communication of basic needs, (3) reading, writing, number concepts, and (4) daily planning. Within each domain is a list of behaviors to consider when evaluating an individual's level of functioning and planning a functional treatment approach. The measure also considers qualitative dimensions of functioning. These include: adequacy (frequency with which the client understands the message); appropriateness (frequency with which the client communicates relevant information); promptness (frequency with which the client responds without delay); and communication sharing (extent to which the client's communication is a burden to the communicative partner).

- This measure was standardized on 185 adults with aphasia or cognitive impairment from 12 geographic regions of the United States.
- The scale is scored from 1 to 7 for communication independence. The scores range from 1 (does not perform even with maximal assistance or prompting) to 4 (does with moderate assistance) to 7 (does with no assistance or prompting).
- A second scale is scored from 1 to 5 for qualitative dimensions. These include ratings for adequacy, appropriateness, promptness, and communication sharing.
- Using the observational rating scale takes approximately 20 minutes.
- A communication independence score is derived.
- Test results are comprehensive and provide meaningful information to the family and help guide rehabilitation services.

Table 2–3 presents the ASHA FACS Framework.

Bedside Assessment

Early in the assessment process, a bedside evaluation may be administered. The Western Aphasia Battery–Revised (WAB-R) (2006) provides a bedside evaluation component that takes approximately 15 minutes to administer. The Bedside Evaluation Screening

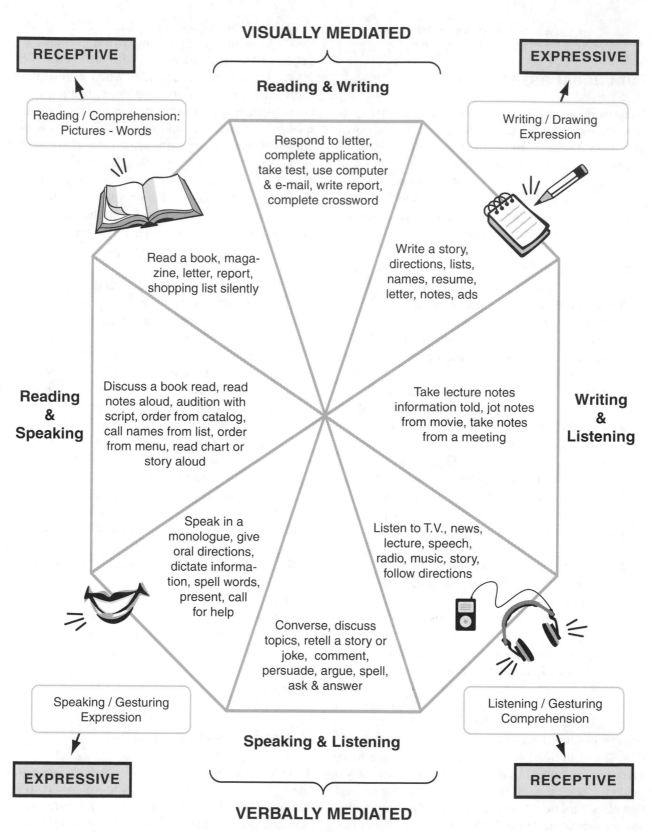

VISUALLY MEDIATED

RECEPTIVE

EXPRESSIVE

Reading & Writing

Reading / Comprehension: Pictures - Words

Writing / Drawing Expression

Respond to letter, complete application, take test, use computer & e-mail, write report, complete crossword

Read a book, magazine, letter, report, shopping list silently

Write a story, directions, lists, names, resume, letter, notes, ads

Reading & Speaking

Discuss a book read, read notes aloud, audition with script, order from catalog, call names from list, order from menu, read chart or story aloud

Take lecture notes information told, jot notes from movie, take notes from a meeting

Writing & Listening

Speak in a monologue, give oral directions, dictate information, spell words, present, call for help

Listen to T.V., news, lecture, speech, radio, music, story, follow directions

Converse, discuss topics, retell a story or joke, comment, persuade, argue, spell, ask & answer

Speaking / Gesturing Expression

Listening / Gesturing Comprehension

Speaking & Listening

EXPRESSIVE

RECEPTIVE

VERBALLY MEDIATED

Figure 2–3. Functional language connections octagon.

Table 2–3. ASHA FACS Framework

Early Assessment

- Introduce yourself to the patient—names can be used to assess verbal memory later.

- Check reading by having the patient read get-well cards and any signs in the room.

- Check the relationship of the person who sent the cards thereby having patient provide a description.

- Ask patient to complete a hospital menu and read what was selected.

- Ask patient to write a few words such as the names of family or friends for word retrieval and writing.

- Ask patient to name a few objects around the room, listening to speech and naming ability.

- Have patient follow a few commands and answer yes/no questions.

- Track higher level comprehension by assessing the patient's ability to track his or her conversation with you. (Holland & Fridriksson, 2001)

Source: Reprinted with permission from *Functional Assessment of Communication Skills for Adults* by C. M. Frattali, A. L. Holland, C. K. Thompson, C. Wohl, and M. Ferketic. Copyright 1995 by American Speech-Language-Hearing Association.

Test (West, Sands, & Ross-Swain, 1998) may help the speech-language pathologist to secure essential language information in a shorter time than other standardized tests. Helm-Estabrooks and Albert (2004) also provide a brief informal exam that may be administered at bedside with the inclusion of several common objects. Areas to assess include: a discourse sample, auditory comprehension skills, naming common objects and coins, repetition of words and sentences, reading printed words, writing names of objects, praxis for individuals who are verbally restricted, and singing a familiar song. Table 2–4 presents sample items for a brief, comprehensive bedside screening tool for aphasia.

Cognition and Aphasia

The person with aphasia has a primary disorder in the area of language; however, we cannot assume that their cognitive functions are normal or con-versely, disordered after the stroke. Cognitive ability plays an important part in daily functioning. Non-brain-injured individuals must engage the world regularly using attention, memory, visuospatial skills, and executive functions combined with language. For example, it is possible that a person who is status post traumatic brain injury (TBI) may be unable to recall information over a brief time span in the presence of normal receptive and expressive language.

Helm-Estabrooks and Albert (2004) indicate that it is faulty to assume that cognition is not affected by a stroke that has produced aphasia. Furthermore, they assert that aphasia may not be "an isolated language disorder." Helm-Estabrooks, Bayles, Ramage, and Bryant (1995) have found that the level of severity of the aphasia is not significantly correlated with the severity of nonverbal cognitive skills. This suggests that cognitive impairment and language impairment after stroke are unique entities that influence one another. Just as attention impacts memory since a person must attend in order to remember information, so do memory skills impact language.

Table 2–4. Sample Items for a Brief, Comprehensive Bedside Screening Tool for Aphasia

Language Functions	Sample Tasks
Basic Auditory Comprehension *Directions:* The clinician gives five commands.	The patient will follow directions and/or manipulate objects from his environment based on clinician instruction: *Ex:* "Hand me your comb." *Ex:* "Point to the door."
Complex Auditory Comprehension *Directions:* The clinician will ask 5 questions about the narrative.	The patient will demonstrate the ability to understand a short narrative presented verbally: *Ex:* "Tell me what happened to X."
Naming *Directions:* The clinician asks the patient to name 5 common objects within his field of vision.	The patient will name objects in his room. *Ex:* "What is this?"
Writing and Functional Word Retrieval *Directions:* The clinician will give the patient paper and pen in order to execute the task.	The patient will write the names of family/friends. *Ex:* "Write the names of your closest family members/friends."
Reading *Directions:* The clinician will locate functional reading material within the patient's room.	The patient will read greeting cards, menu, and newspapers available in his room. *Ex:* "Read this greeting card to me."
Expressive Language *Directions:* The clinician asks leading questions to facilitate expressive language.	The patient will describe a room of his house: *Ex:* "Describe your bedroom at home for me."
Repetition *Directions:* The clinician asks the client to repeat words, phrases, and sentences of increasing length.	The patient will repeat a word/phrase/sentence: *Ex:* "Repeat each word or phrase after me: book, my big book, I want my big book."
Verbal memory *Directions:* Upon entering the room and greeting the patient, the clinician will offer his/her name.	The patient will remember the clinician's name once introduced. *Ex:* "I gave you my name three minutes ago. What is my name?"
Reasoning/Judgment *Directions:* The clinician can choose to develop the question from any home-based safety scenarios.	The patient will respond to a home-based scenario: *Ex:* "What would you do if you ran out of a very important medicine?"
Speech/Voice *Directions:* The clinician will monitor the patient's voice for quality, pitch, resonance, respiration and loudness and articulatory accuracy and speech intelligibility.	The patient will produce an automatic speech sequence: *Ex:* "Name the days of the week."

Directions for Use: Use this beside screening instrument to delineate deficit areas. The clinician can then determine the most appropriate diagnostic instrument to administer in order to provide further clinical insights into the patient's communication profile. This would optimize treatment planning and goal selection.

The general principle is that the cognitive functions listed above interact and influence reading, writing, listening, and speaking, depending on the task. In normal functioning individuals, it is difficult to imagine a person holding a meaningful conversation without the ability to attend and use information stored in memory. Professionals working with people with aphasia would be remiss if they did not consider a patient's ability to attend to tasks, use memory functions, perceive visuospatial details, and engage their executive functions. We suggest that clinicians screen these areas of cognitive ability using nonverbal measures such as the Cognitive Linguistic Quick Test (CLQT) (Helm-Estabrooks, 2001) or the Cognitive Linguistic Evaluation (Appendix C).

In patients with cognitive deficits, the clinician must address those therapeutically before or in conjunction with language therapy (Helm-Estabrooks & Albert, 2004). Consider the task of trail making. In this activity the client must attend to circles and triangles interspersed randomly on a page. Specifically, the task is to draw a line from a circle to a triangle keeping that pattern until all the shapes are connected. Such a nonverbal task requires general attentional skills, sequential memory, and visuospatial ability. Once the clinician has obtained the results, a therapy plan for the patient must incorporate this information. For instance, if the clinician plans to use a therapy program such as Melodic Intonation Therapy (MIT) (Helm-Estabrooks & Albert, 2004, p. 221) or the Sentence Production Program for Aphasia (SPPA) (Helm-Estabrooks & Albert, 2004, p. 235) which requires attention to black and white line drawings, it is necessary to consider information about their visuospatial skills. This will impact the patient's success and may require the clinician to select other stimuli. Without a cognitive screening and/or evaluation, the clinician may miss vital details to support the patient's success.

Cognitive Examination in Acquired Language Disorders

As noted above, cognitive ability plays an important part in daily functioning. For people who have cognitive-linguistic deficits, operating within the world is challenging due to their impaired language, attention, memory, executive functions, and/or visuospatial abilities. Once the clinician has obtained a thorough case history of the person with aphasia, we believe that the most important aspects of cognition to be addressed are:

- Attention
- Memory
- Language
- Executive functions
- Visuospatial skills

Attention

The ability to pay attention has important therapeutic implications, that is, attending to tasks within the therapy session. In addition, attention is of primary importance if one is to be safe and interactive in the environment. Therefore, we suggest that the clinician determine if the patient demonstrates *vigilance*, which is the ability to maintain attention over time. The underlying abilities necessary for vigilance are obviously being awake and alert. The patient must also be able to shift attention as needed, that is, demonstrate *selective attention*. This is an important cognitive skill that is necessary for success in therapy as well as for the individual to participate in social life and in their environment. The clinician must also evaluate the patient's ability to plan and multitask, which include examples of *executive attention*. In order to live independently or with minimal supervision, a patient must be able to plan their daily activities and manage information and situations that may happen simultaneously, typically an everyday occurrence. Two very simple methods of testing attention are using symbol cancellation tasks and trail-making tasks. Both require the patient to maintain attention (vigilance), shift attention continuously (selective attention), and plan their next move (executive attention). Many cognitive workbooks include these types of tasks and clinicians can devise their own.

Memory

In general, there are three types of cognitive memory (memory requiring thought). They are called episodic, working, and semantic memory. *Episodic memory* is used when we are remembering our own past experiences and events that we have participated in throughout the day. Evaluating this aspect of cognitive memory can help the clinician with a differential diagnosis (e.g., raising questions about one's ability to recall events, which is important to know in assessing for dementia). For example, the patient may benefit from a memory book to assist with planning and keeping appointments. *Working memory* is necessary for normal conversation. An individual must have the ability to retrieve words to express their thoughts and retain the content of the other speaker's information in order to respond appropriately. People with aphasia may lack the working memory necessary to engage in discourse. The ability to sequence information and hold it in memory for processing and manipulation is a complex task requiring several systems to work simultaneously. *Semantic memory* is the storehouse for our conceptual knowledge of the world and for factual information that we have learned. It is obvious that a patient with an impaired semantic memory will be at a severe disadvantage due to their inability to retrieve facts and concepts pertinent to activities of daily living.

In addition to the more cognitive domains of memory, *procedural memory* is used during execution of automatic tasks that were previously learned by the patient and therefore often considered noncognitive in nature. In the aphasic patient, the clinician must determine if procedural memory has been affected by the neurologic event in case she wants to use any of those previously learned tasks in therapy. Consulting with the occupational therapist (OT) is recommended during in an evaluation in order to eventually co-treat the patient optimally. The OT can assess and treat the patient's functional capabilities for activities of daily living, giving the speech-language pathologist (SLP) insight into the patient's procedural memory for those tasks. This can help the SLP with functional goal formulation.

Language

The relationship between language and cognition is intricate and well-established. Any comprehensive diagnostic language instrument designed to evaluate the person with aphasia should include the following linguistic areas for assessment:

- Semantics
- Syntax
- Morphology
- Pragmatics
- Phonology

Cognition is dealt with in more detail in the following chapters on the aphasic syndromes. However, we believe that the ability to compensate for one's language deficits must take into account one's cognitive skills. The extent of damage to the patient's cognition will influence therapeutic considerations. Areas assessed in a comprehensive cognitive-linguistic evaluation typically include the following:

- Perception
- Discrimination
- Orientation/awareness
- Organization of thoughts
- Memory (immediate/recent/long-term)
- Reasoning/problem-solving/inference
- Auditory processing and comprehension
- Calculation
- Reading and visual processing
- Writing
- Pragmatics and affect

Executive Functions

Executive functions refer to the highest level of human cognitive ability. It is very possible to sustain significant language impairment secondary to stroke and still have intact executive functions. The patient may simply not be able to demonstrate this to the clinician verbally. Therefore, assessing executive functions nonverbally must be considered in the person with aphasia. Executive functions include tasks such as *planning*, *sequencing*, *accomplishing goal-directed behavior*, *maintaining flexibility*, *problem-solving*, *reasoning*, and *judgment*. These skills are needed in order to function independently in the world. Evaluating these skills will help the clinician in post-discharge planning by informing other team members of cognitive assessment outcomes. Furthermore, the status of a patient's executive functioning will impact selection of language goals. Some tests that the SLP can use to evaluate this area include the Wisconsin Card Sorting Test (Psychological Assessment Resources,

2003), Tower of Hanoi, and/or the Maze Solving subtest from the Cognitive Linguistic Quick Test (CLQT).

Visuospatial Skills

Visuospatial skills must be assessed in order to know if any confrontation naming deficits, writing and/or reading problems are affected by this type of impairment. The clinician must evaluate the patient's visual fields to rule out visual inattention, visual neglect, or a visual field cut due to hemianopsia. The occupational therapist will also be invaluable for consultation in this area. *Visual perception* encompasses the ability to discriminate, analyze, recognize, and interpret visual stimuli. Visual perception is an extremely important skill when working with the aphasic patient as the SLP tends to use visual stimuli to facilitate language production. Another visuospatial skill necessary for language therapy is *visual construction*. This is defined as the ability to combine visual perception with a motor response. This skill is critical for writing, printing and drawing which in some cases remains the only functional communication modality in people with aphasia. Both the Rey Complex Figure Test (Myers & Myers, 1995) and the Boston Assessment of Severe Aphasia (BASA) (Helm-Estabrooks, Ramsberger, & Nichols, 1989) assess some of these skills.

Integrating Tasks: Clock Drawing. The clock-drawing task has been used for many years as a quick but very effective tool in the assessment of cognition in the person with aphasia. Why? Here is the instruction:

> *Draw a clock, put in all the numbers, and set the clock to 10 minutes after 11.*

In order to complete this task, the patient must possess the *language skills* to process the directions and write the numbers in the correct place on a clock. He must have the *memory* to store and later retrieve the time setting. He must have the *visuospatial skills* to represent the clock correctly. He must possess *visuoperceptual attention*, and motor skills to execute the mental image. Finally, he must have the *executive functions* that are needed to plan the task and make adjustments if necessary. In short, *clock drawing* enables the speech-language pathologist to get a glimpse of the patient's cognitive skills to plan therapeutically.

Use of Standardized Tests for Individuals with Cognitive-Communication Disorders

It is a challenge to assess individuals with cognitive-communication disorders. The Academy of Neurologic Communication Disorders and Sciences (ANCDS) has written on the topic of use of standardized, norm-referenced tests for individuals with cognitive-communication disorders (Turkstra, Coelho, & Ylvisaker, 2005). A committee analyzed the use of performance measures and questionnaires regarding strengths and limitations. Reliability and validity were also important factors in consideration of appropriate tests. Four key questions for test evaluation included: (1) Does the person have a problem? (2) If there is a cognitive-communication disorder, what are the characteristics? (3) What are the implications of the test results beyond the test session? and (4) Where should I begin with treatment? For a complete list of the standardized tests that were reviewed, see Turkstra, Coelho, and Ylvisaker (2005). Of the 32 assessment measures reviewed, the following seven tests met most of the criteria for standardized assessment of individuals with cognitive-communication disorders:

- American Speech-Language-Hearing Association Functional Assessment of Communication Skills in Adults (ASHA FACS) (Frattali, Thompson, Holland, Wohl, & Ferketic, 1995)
- Behavior Rating Inventory of Executive Function (BRIEF) (Gioia, Isquith, Guy, & Kenworthy, 2000)
- Communication Activities of Daily Living, Second Edition (CADL-2) (Holland, Frattali, & Fromm, 1999)
- Functional Independence Measure (FIM, 1996; Uniform Data System for Medical Rehabilitation)

■ Repeatable Battery for the Assessment of Neuropsychological Status (RBANS) (Randolph, 2001)
■ Test of Language Competence-Extended (TLC-E) (Wiig & Secord, 1989)
■ Western Aphasia Battery (WAB) (Kertesz, 1982), updated to the WAB-Revised (Kertesz, 2006)

Commonly Used Assessments for Acquired Language Disorders: Key Concepts and Information

The assessment measures listed below are frequently used to assess individuals with aphasia and cognitive-communication disorders. Details regarding testing purpose, appropriateness for patient types, standardization information, and administration factors are included.

Burns Brief Inventory of Communication and Cognition (Burns, 1997)

The Burns is designed for adults with neurologic impairment.

■ It assesses individuals with
  ■ Left hemisphere focal lesions
  ■ Right hemisphere focal lesions
  ■ Complex neuropathologies
■ Assesses specific skills a patient has and their level of functioning.
■ Determines if individuals with left hemisphere lesions have language deficits consistent with aphasia
■ Determines if individuals with right hemisphere lesions have patterns of aprosodia (lack of speech prosody) or visuospatial cognitive deficits consistent with right hemisphere syndrome
■ Determines if individuals with head injury or early dementing diseases have attention

and memory problems consistent with these disease processes
■ Its scoring is set up to help determine what areas to treat first (scored areas falling within the shaded zones are optimal for initial treatment).
■ It is standardized on individuals from 18 to 80 years and is to be administered by speech-language pathologists.
■ Reliability and validity studies have been completed with adequate results found.
■ It is easy to administer and score—each inventory (3 total) takes about 30 minutes.
■ Differential scoring is considered for repetition, self-correction, cueing, or delayed responses

Western Aphasia Battery—Revised (WAB-R) (Kertesz, 2006)

The WAB-R is designed for differential diagnosis of English-speaking adults and teens with neurologic disorders.

■ It assesses individuals with: stroke, head injury, and dementia.
■ It contains a bedside evaluation as a screening tool that takes 15 minutes.
■ It contains a comprehensive evaluation comprised of 8 subtests with oral/verbal sections taking 30 to 45 minutes and reading sections taking 45 to 60 minutes.
■ It provides diagnostic information about linguistic and key nonlinguistic skills most frequently affected by aphasia.
■ It provides an Aphasia Quotient, Cortical Quotient, Auditory Comprehension Quotient, Oral Expression Quotient, Reading Quotient, Writing Quotient, and bedside WAB-R scores based on 32 short tasks.
■ Areas tested include: content, fluency, auditory comprehension, repetition, naming, word finding, reading, writing, drawing, block design, calculation, and praxis.
■ It contains statistical research with evidence of reliability and validity along

with information about its use for people with head injury and dementia.

- The WAB-R is considered a good predictor of patients' vocational outcomes.
- The test can be administered in sections and it gives a comprehensive aphasia classification (Global, Broca's, Isolation, Transcortical Motor, Wernicke's, Transcortical Sensory, Conduction, and Anomic).
- It has been standardized on 150 patients with aphasia and 59 control subjects.
- The test booklet provides an outline for each section and provides details linking scores with aphasia types

The Cognitive Linguistic Quick Test (Helm-Estabrooks, 2001)

The CLQT is a criterion-referenced test for English and Spanish-speaking adults with acquired neurologic dysfunction.

- It assesses individuals with deficits affecting:
  - Attention
  - Memory
  - Language
  - Visuospatial skills
  - Executive dysfunction
- Assesses strengths and weaknesses of the 5 cognitive domains: attention, memory, language, visuospatial skills, and executive functions.
- Used to identify cognitive strengths and weaknesses.
- It is not considered a comprehensive tool for differential diagnosis.
- Patients must be able to use a pen and give verbal responses to take this test.
- More abstract items may require a professional with experience for interpretation and application.
- It provides a performance review of cognitive abilities affecting functioning.
- The test takes approximately 30 minutes to administer.

Communicative Activities of Daily Living-2 (Holland, Frattali, & Fromm, 1999)

The CADL-2 is designed for adults with neurogenic disorders.

- It assesses functional communication skills of:
  - Reading
  - Writing
  - Using numbers
  - Social interaction
  - Context utilization
  - Role-playing
  - Sequential relationships
  - Divergences
  - Nonverbal communication
- This test was standardized on 175 individuals 20 to 96 years old with neurologically based communication disorders across 17 states in the United States.
- The test provides information about the patient's communication strategies, pragmatic skills, and interaction abilities that are functional in nature.
- Areas assessed include greetings, answering questions, and performing activities of daily living such as ordering from a menu, reading a bus schedule, determining what to do next in a given situation, completing forms, matching symbols with pictures, making plans and scheduling, to name several.
- It can also be used for individuals with mental retardation, dementia, traumatic brain injury, and right hemisphere syndrome.
- It contains 50 items and is generally administered in 30 to 50 minutes by a licensed, certified speech-language pathologist.
- Patients can ask for repetition of items.
- Video recording is encouraged for assessing nonverbal as well as verbal behaviors.
- Differential scoring is provided for adequacy of responses.

■ Results can pinpoint strengths in communication and determine what the patient is functionally able to communicate.

Ross Information Processing Assessment-2 (Ross-Swain, 1996)

The RIPA-2 is designed for individuals 15 to 90 years old with neurogenic disorders.

■ It assesses:
  ■ Memory
  ■ Orientation
  ■ Organization
  ■ Reasoning
  ■ Auditory processing
■ The RIPA-2 was developed as an efficient, standardized test that quantifies and qualifies cognitive-linguistic deficits.
■ The subtests assess aspects of memory, orientation, recall of information, problem solving, abstract reasoning, organizational ability, auditory processing, and retention.
■ Scoring is based on a 3-point system which considers intelligibility, perseveration, confabulation, and tangential information as errors.
■ The test requires minimal materials and is easy to administer.
■ Scoring requires use of different diacritical markers.
■ Reliability and validity studies have been performed on individuals with TBI (traumatic brain injury).

Scales of Cognitive Ability for Traumatic Brain Injury (Adamovich & Henderson, 1992)

The SCATBI is designed for patients with acquired brain damage.

■ It assesses cognitive deficits associated with TBI including:

■ Perception and discrimination (including attention)
■ Orientation
■ Organization
■ Recall
■ Reasoning
■ This measure assesses cognitive-linguistic status during recovery from head injury and measures the extent of change during a program of rehabilitation.
■ The test was standardized on head-injured patients throughout the United States and Canada. The subjects ranged from 15 years to 88 years old.
■ The SCATBI provides a systematic method to assess cognitive deficits.
■ Test items are arranged with increasing difficulty.
■ Administration takes approximately 2 hours with each section taking from 10 to 45 minutes, ranging from lower to higher difficulty levels.
■ The five scales of the SCATBI are: perception/discrimination, orientation, organization, recall, and reasoning. Items include: Initiating, sustaining, and shifting attention, discriminating between shapes and sounds, knowing time, place, and setting, grouping and sequencing based on rules, recalling information from semantic memory and episodic memory with immediate, delayed, and long-term memory stores, and inductive and deductive reasoning.
■ Within each section there are tests to determine the patient's cognitive abilities. These comprise 40 testlets.
■ Minimal materials are needed to administer the test and the testlets can be given separately.
■ The instructions are clear. Stimulus cards and the manual must be used simultaneously.
■ A severity score is determined from the patient's overall performance. Scores can reflect an initial level and patient progress with readministered throughout the patient's recovery.

Arizona Battery for Communication Disorders of Dementia (Bayles & Tomoeda, 1993)

The ABCD is designed for patients with neurologic disorders including dementia and head injury.

- It assesses:
  - Linguistic expression
  - Linguistic comprehension
  - Verbal episodic memory
  - Visuospatial construction
  - Mental status
- The ABCD was designed to identify and describe information about nonlinguistic and linguistic communication deficits in dementia.
- The ABCD was standardized on patients with Alzheimer's disease and Parkinson's disease as well as young and older healthy individuals.
- The ABCD allows clinicians to have an understanding of the patient's mental status and their ability to read, name, describe, define, repeat, answer questions, follow directions, retell a story, recall and recognize words, copy figures, and draw.
- There are 14 primary subtests in the ABCD. These include:

  Mental status, story retelling, following commands, comparative questions, word learning (free recall, total recall, recognition), repetition, object description, reading comprehension (word and sentence levels), generative naming, confrontation naming, concept definition, generative drawing, figure copying, and story retelling (delayed).
- The test is easy to administer and score. Single subtests can be used.
- Test responses can aid clinicians in planning intervention strategies.
- Testing the full battery takes from 45 to 90 minutes.
- Test results help determine how coherent the patient is to the environment and how well he/she is able to follow directions,

compare information to make judgments, and recognize and identify uses for objects that are common in the home.

Boston Diagnostic Aphasia Examination-3 (Goodglass, Kaplan, & Barresi, 2001)

The BDAE-3 is designed for assessing patients with aphasia.

- It assesses the nature of deficits for:
  - Auditory comprehension
  - Articulation
  - Fluency
  - Word finding
  - Repetition
  - Serial speech
  - Grammar and syntax
  - Paraphasia
- The BDAE-3 is a diagnostic test to diagnose the presence and type of aphasic syndrome, to measure performance of a wide range of abilities, and to provide a comprehensive assessment of the patient's strengths and weaknesses in language areas in order to guide treatment.
- The test has both long and short forms and also includes the Boston Naming Test to assess lexical retrieval abilities.
- The test assesses five areas of functioning: conversational and expository speech, auditory comprehension, oral expression, reading, and writing.

  Testing of conversational and expository speech includes simple social responses, free conversation, picture description, and narrative discourse. It provides a severity rating and speech output characteristics profile. Auditory comprehension testing assesses word comprehension, following commands of increasing complexity, understanding complex ideational material, and syntactic processing with comprehension of embedded sentences. Oral expression is assessed for oral agility, automatic sequences, recitation, melody and rhythm, repetition abilities, and naming. Reading is assessed for basic symbol recognition, word identification, phonics, derivational and grammatical morphology, and oral reading with comprehension of words, sentences, and paragraphs. Writing assessment includes mechanics, writing to dictation, oral spelling, written picture naming, grammar, and narrative writing. Praxis is also tested for limb and hand as well as for buccofacial and respiratory abilities.

■ Using the rating scale profile form, the type of aphasic syndrome can be identified with a degree of validity.

■ The test was standardized on 85 aphasic subjects from inpatient, outpatient, and private practice sources with a range of severity ratings and 15 normal elderly volunteers.

Psycholinguistic Assessments of Language Processing in Aphasia (Kay, Lesser, & Coltheart, 1992)

The PALPA is designed for patients with acquired brain damage and aphasia.

■ It assesses language processing and evaluates:
  ■ Recognition
  ■ Comprehension
  ■ Production of spoken words and sentences
  ■ Production of written words and sentences
■ The PALPA consists of 60 assessments to help diagnose language processing difficulties in people with acquired brain damage.
■ Subtest areas are selected according to the patient's individualized needs.
■ The battery is divided intro four primary areas: (1) Auditory Processing, (2) Reading and Spelling, (3) Picture and Word Semantics, and (4) Sentence

Comprehension. Modules include recognizing printed words, understanding printed words, reading aloud, recognizing objects and pictures, recognizing and repeating speech, spelling, writing, sentence processing, and more.

■ Data was obtained on 25 subjects with aphasia and 32 nonbrain-damaged subjects, matched for age, education, and social variables. Descriptive statistical analyses (means and standard deviations) are provided as a gauge for abnormal performance.

■ The materials provided may also be used for a variety of procedures and tasks.

■ This lengthy test has studies reporting on its use. See *Aphasiology: An International, Interdisciplinary Journal, 18*(2), from February, 2004.

Cognitive Linguistic Evaluation (Shipley & McAfee, 2004)

This informal tool is comprehensive in its range of content and provides an overview of cognitive-linguistic skills of adults and teens.

■ It assesses:
  ■ Perception
  ■ Discrimination
  ■ Orientation/awareness
  ■ Organization of thoughts
  ■ Memory (immediate/recent/long-term)
  ■ Reasoning/problem-solving/inference
  ■ Auditory processing and comprehension
  ■ Calculation
  ■ Reading and visual processing
  ■ Writing
  ■ Pragmatics and affect

The area of cognitive-linguistics developed from the field of linguistics with an understanding that language development and language use are best explained in reference to human cognition. In the area of cognitive linguistic study there are three primary premises: (1) there is no autonomous linguistic faculty in one's mind, (2) grammar is a conceptualization, and (3) knowledge of language comes from language use (Croft & Cruse, 2004). Cognitive-linguistic evaluations typically include knowledge that addresses the following types of items:

- Orientation to the date, time, season, where someone lives and for how long, one's name, profession, and additional items as pertient to the individual.
- Memory for recall of numbers and words, retelling a story, indicating food eaten during the day, activities of the day, where born, birth date, family members' names, and additional facts.
- Auditory processing and comprehension involving yes-no questions for basic information including one's name and residence, answering yes/no questions for factual and abstract information.
- Problem-solving for questions given situations, logic and reasoning, inferential knowledge for correcting illogical statements, providing meanings for common expressions and proverbs, naming items given a series of clues, and indicating categories for similar items.
- Thought organization for providing definitions of words, steps taken to accomplish tasks, and planning strategies in addition to higher level tasks pertinent to the individual.
- Calculation for numerical word problems involving quantities, money, and time.
- Reading and visual processing for reading words and determining ones that do not belong in the group, following a series of written directions, reading sentences aloud and answering questions about a paragraph, telling time from clock drawings, and attending to specific shapes on a page.
- Writing one's name and date, writing a short description of activities accomplished during the day, and other written work pertinent to the individual.
- Pragmatic behaviors of language including appropriateness of physical proximity,

eye contact and facial expression, use of gestures, prosody, topic maintenance, turn-taking, initiation, attention, organization, and ability to limit distractibility

Appendix C (Cognitive Linguistic Evaluation) presents the cognitive-linguistic evaluation.

Treatment and Goal Setting

Working with patients within a rehabilitation framework requires the SLP to consider the patient's individual needs and desires while simultaneously considering their level of impairments and functional abilities. Family members, friends, and significant others are excellent resources in establishing appropriate goals. The goals of treatment in therapy should always meet the following criteria:

- Promote function.
- Promote an effective communicative environment.
- Provide compensatory strategies to communicate if a return to the patient's premorbid communication status is not possible or feasible.
- Provide education and counseling for adjustment of the patient and family
- Reduce interfering behaviors.
- Provide a relevant home program to the patient and family.

Documentation of Progress

It is essential to continually record progress regarding the patient's performance of therapeutic tasks. For example, the following note may be developed:

- Pt. (patient) obtained 38% accuracy for 8 targets (3/8) in 3 minutes on 1/5/09 and reached 88% accuracy for 16 targets (14/16) in 2 minutes on 2/5/09.
- Family log noted greater attention to visual details.

■ Pt. read all words in a sentence given a local newspaper.

Writing progress is often accomplished using SOAP Notes. The acronym S.O.A.P. reflects the following:

■ **S**ubjective—general impressions of the client during the session (feelings and statements about the client from the client and/or the family are given, information about the client's behavior during the session may be written, and factors that may have affected the client's progress or lack of progress may be included in this section).
■ **O**bjective—measurable information about the treatment, indicating the behavioral objectives (data that is quantitative and/or qualitative, behavioral objective(s) and current data are written in this section).
■ **A**ssessment—an analysis of the session with objective findings, interpretation of results of the session reflecting if the client is making progress (indicate if the client is making progress in therapy, provide a cohesive statement, indicate if performance has improved, declined, or remained the same with factors that may be contributing).
■ **P**lan—the course of treatment and plans are provided in this section. (provide a logical follow-up to the previous section on assessment, indicate what is next).

A sample SOAP note:

S: Patient appeared alert and cooperative. He said, "I'm ready to work today!"

O: Pt. followed one-step commands at 80% accuracy with visual and verbal cues given 20 trials.

A: Withdrawal of visual cues (hand gestures) resulted in a decrease of accurate direction following down to 40% for one-step commands.

P: Continue therapy twice weekly. Include family member in session, if possible.

Continue current treatment tasks with verbal cues however reduce visual cues systematically by intermittently using hand gestures.

Functional Goals

Suggested functional activities are listed in Figure 2–3. This partial list of activities further illustrates the many reading-writing-listening-speaking connections individuals engage in during activities of daily living. Both verbal (listening and speaking) and visual (reading and writing) modalities must be considered when planning functional treatments for patients. It is important not to frustrate the patient but as treatment professionals we want to provide them with meaningful tasks to enhance their quality of life.

References

Adamovich, B. L. B., & Henderson, J. (1992). *Scales of cognitive ability for traumatic brain injury.* Chicago: Riverside.

Bayles, K. A., & Tomoeda, C. K. (1993). *Arizona battery of communication disorders of dementia (ABCD).* Austin, TX: Pro-Ed.

Burns, M. (1997). *Burns brief inventory of communication and cognition.* San Antonio, TX: Psychological Corporation.

Caplan, D. (1987). *Neurolinguistics and linguistic aphasiology.* Cambridge, UK: Cambridge University Press.

Croft, W., & Cruse, D. A. (2004). *Cognitive linguistics.* Cambridge, UK: Cambridge University Press.

Frattali, C., Thompson, C., Holland, A., Wohl, C., & Ferketic, M. (1995). *American speech-language-hearing association functional assessment of communication skills for adults.* Rockville, MD: American Speech-Language-Hearing Association.

Functional Independence Measure. (1996). *Uniform data set for medical rehabilitation.* Buffalo, NY: University of Buffalo.

Gioia, G. A., Isquith, P. K., Guy, S. C., & Kenworthy, L. (2000). *Behavior rating inventory of executive function.* Odessa, FL: Psychological Assessment Resources.

Goodglass, H., Kaplan, E., & Barresi, B. (2001). *The Boston diagnostic aphasia exam.* Philadelphia: Lippincott Williams & Wilkins

Helm-Estabrooks, N. (2001). *Cognitive linguistic quick test*. San Antonio, TX: Psychological Corporation.

Helm-Estabrooks, N., & Albert, M. (1991). *Manual of aphasia therapy*. Austin, TX: Pro-Ed.

Helm-Estabrooks, N., & Albert, M. L. (2004). *Manual of aphasia and aphasia therapy* (2nd ed.). Austin, TX: Pro-Ed.

Helm-Estabrooks, N., Bayles K., Ramage, A., & Bryant, S. (1995). Relationship between cognitive performance and aphasia severity, age, and education: Females versus males. *Brain and Language, 51*(1), 139–141.

Helm-Estabrooks, N., Ramsberger, A. R., & Nichols, M. (1989). *Boston assessment of severe aphasia*. Dedham, MA: AliMed.

Holland, A., Frattali, C., & Fromm, D. (1999). *Communication activities of daily living* (2nd ed.). Austin, TX: Pro-Ed.

Holland, A., & Fridriksson, J. (2001). Aphasia management during the early phases of recovery following stroke. *American Journal of Speech-Language Pathology, 10*, 19–28.

Kay, J., Lesser, R., & Coltheart, R. M. (1992). *Psycholinguistic assessments of language processing in aphasia*. Hove, East Sussex, UK: Lawrence Erlbaum.

Kertesz, A. (2006). *Western Aphasia Battery-Revised*. San Antonio, TX. Psychological Corporation.

Klein, E. R., & Hahn, S. E. (2007). *Focus on function: Gaining essential communication* (2nd ed.). Austin, TX: Pro-Ed.

Kohn, S. (1989). The nature of the phonemic string deficit in conduction aphasia. *Aphasiology, 3*, 265–285.

Kohn, S. (1993). Segmental disorders in aphasia. In G. Blanken, J. Dittmann, H. Grimm, J. Marshall, & C. W. Wallesch (Eds.), *Linguistic disorders and pathologies: An international handbook* (pp. 197–209). Berlin: Walter de Gruyter.

Meyers, J. E., & Meyers, K. R. (1995). *Rey Complex Figure Test and Recognition Trial*. San Antonio, TX: Pearson Education.

Psychological Assessment Resources. (2003). *The Wisconsin Card Sorting Test: Computerized Version 4 (WCST)*. Lutz, FL: Psychological Assessment Resources.

Randolph, C. (2001). *Repeatable battery for the assessment of neuropsychological status*. San Antonio, TX: Psychological Corporation.

Ross-Swain, D. (1996). *Ross Information Processing Assessment* (2nd ed.). Austin, TX: Pro-Ed.

Shipley, K. G., & McAfee, J. G. (2004). *Assessment in speech-language pathology: A resource manual*. (3rd ed.) Clifton Park, NY: Delmar

Turkstra, L. S., Coelho, C., & Ylvisaker, M. (2005). The use of standardized tests for individuals with cognitive-communication disorders. *Seminars in Speech and Language, 26*(4), 215–222.

West, J. F., Sands, E., & Ross-Swain, D. (1998). *Bedside Evaluation Screening Test*. Austin, TX: Pro-Ed.

Wiig, E., & Secord, W. (1989). *Test of Language Competence—Expanded Edition*. San Antonio, TX: Psychological Corporation.

Chapter 3

THE MAJOR NONFLUENT APHASIAS

Broca's Aphasia

Characteristics

Individuals who have a Broca's aphasia are nonfluent. Their speech is effortful, imprecisely articulated, and their melodic line, or prosody, ranges from aprosodic to normal intonation contours in short phrases (Basso, 2003). Even though the person with a Broca's aphasia is nonfluent, they are able to repeat, although with varying difficulty (Basso, 2003). The articulation deficit is generally considered by most researchers and clinicians to be apraxia of speech (Rosenbeck et al., 1989). The person with a Broca's aphasia generally uses simplified grammar that does not include function words or morphemes and consists mainly of nouns. This renders their output agrammatic (Basso, 2003; Davis, 2007; Thompson, 2008). In some individuals, verbal output may not extend beyond the word level. An individual with a nonfluent aphasia tends to be more fluent when producing automatic sequences, that is, counting, days of the week, and months of the year.

Anomia is also a predominant feature of Broca's aphasia (Basso, 2003). An interesting feature of this impairment is that the ease of word finding is proportional to verbal fluency. For example, if the individual is limited in verbal output, word finding tends to be more impaired. In addition, auditory comprehension is usually mildly or moderately impaired (Basso, 2003; Davis, 2007); however, in lengthy paragraphs or when there are multiple speakers in a conversational context, comprehension can be further compromised. People with Broca's aphasia can be effective communicators because the words they are able to produce do have semantic content, and the listener can fill in the blanks based on context (Davis, 2007).

The presence of motor speech disorders, that is, apraxia of speech and dysarthria, in a person with Broca's aphasia is common, further complicating the speaker's ability to communicate effectively. A mild dysarthria typically is observed; however, if apraxia of speech is also present, the person's speech intelligibility may be more compromised due to the interaction of these two speech disorders (LaPointe, 2005). Despite the general constellation of features common to a particular type of communication disorder, the clinician must keep in mind that patient variability is high in neurogenic impairments. Consequently, level of severity is always a factor in the clinical presentation of a particular patient, that is, a mild dysarthria may be the general case, but a particular patient may present with more significant impairment, if even for a short time.

Broca's aphasia was historically attributed to a lesion in Broca's area. Figure 3–1 shows Brodmann's areas 44 and 45. This area is located at the foot of the inferior frontal gyrus within the third frontal convolution of the left hemisphere, which receives its blood supply from the left middle cerebral artery (LMCA) (see Figure 3–1). However, it is now recognized that damage to this area does not produce a *frank* Broca's aphasia. Instead, the observed deficits include a mild dysarthria with dysprosody and a mild

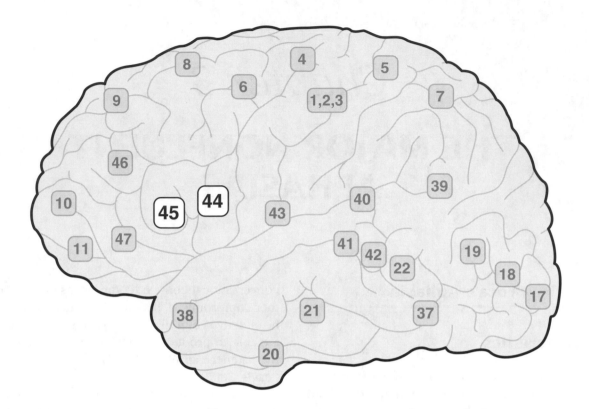

Areas 1, 2 & 3 - Primary Somatosensory Cortex
Area 4 - Primary Motor Cortex
Area 5 - Somatosensory Association Cortex
Area 6 - Pre-Motor and Supplementary Motor Cortex
Area 7 - Somatosensory Association Cortex
Area 8 - Includes frontal eye fields
Area 9 - Dorsolateral prefrontal cortex
Area 10 - Frontopolar area
Area 11 - Orbitofrontal area
Area 17 - Primary Visual Cortex (V1)
Area 18 - Visual Association Cortex (V2)
Area 19 - V3
Area 20 - Inferior Temporal gyrus

Area 21 - Middle Temporal gyrus
Area 22 - Superior Temporal gyrus
Area 37 - Fusiform gyrus
Area 38 - Temporopolar area
Area 39 - Angular gyrus, part of Wernicke's area
Area 40 - Supramarginal gyrus part of Wernicke's area
Areas 41 & 42 - Primary and Auditory Association Cortex
Area 43 - Subcentral area
        (between insula and post/precentral gyrus)
Area 44 - Pars opercularis (part of Broca's area)
Area 45 - Pars triangularis Broca's area
Area 46 - Dorsolateral prefrontal cortex
Area 47 - Inferior prefrontal gyrus

Figure 3–1. Brodmann's areas.

agraphia, that is, difficult writing. Current imaging techniques have revealed that a *chronic* Broca's aphasia results from sizable damage to the frontal operculum and the insula. More specifically, a frank Broca's aphasia results from a large lesion and includes the left lateral frontal suprasylvian, pre-Rolandic region (Johnson & Jacobson, 2007). This lesion also extends into the periventricular white matter, some tracts of the posterior internal capsule, and often includes the inferior parietal lobe (Davis, 2007). Notably, in the *acute phase* of the stroke, a much smaller infarct is needed to produce a typical Broca's aphasia.

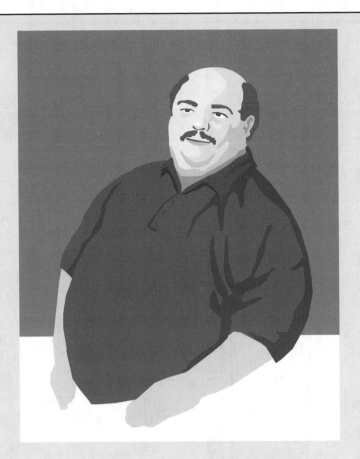

Case Scenario: Maurice

History and Physical (H & P): 48 yrs., white male, right-handed, admitted via Emergency Department with stroke in progress characterized by "slurred speech" and right upper extremity weakness.

Past Medical History (PMH): Insulin-Dependent Diabetes Mellitus Type II (IDDM), hypertension (HTN), morbidly obese, carotid artery occlusion bilaterally, worse on left.

Social History: Married; two children (22 yrs. and 19 yrs.); insurance salesman; lives with wife.

Surgical History: s/p (status post) appendectomy.

A Functional Analysis of Maurice

Maurice's expressive language skills are the most significantly impaired of his language functions (see Maurice's deficits under Case Analysis). Reading comprehension and auditory comprehension approximated normal; however, at more

Category	Findings
Language Expression	**Automatic Speech:** None; attempts characterized by vowel sounds.
	Repetition Ability: Fair at monosyllabic level.
	Lexical Retrieval-Naming: Unable to determine secondary to sparse, non-fluent output.
	Conversational Ability: Agrammatic; unable to converse.
	Pragmatic Skills: Social gestures used appropriately.
	Paraphasias: None.
Speech	**Rate:** Cannot determine due to non-fluent speech.
	Intelligibility: Beyond monosyllables, intelligibility is poor secondary to apraxia of speech.
	Prosody: Intonation contours observed in phrases such as oh, boy!
	Articulation: Substitutions, omissions predominate; distortions noted secondary to unilateral upper motor neuron (UMN) dysarthria.
	Fluency: Poor.
Auditory Comprehension	**Answering Yes/No Questions:** Very good for concrete/personal content.
	Executing Commands: within functional limits (WFL)
	Understanding Stories & Paragraphs: Good at paragraph level.
	Understanding Conversational Speech: WFL; group settings pose some difficulty.
	Identifying Objects & their Functions: WFL
Reading	**Word-level Comprehension:** Good.
	Sentence-level Comprehension: Good at paragraph level with concrete information.
	Oral Reading: Unable to assess secondary to severity of apraxia of speech.
	Oral Spelling: Unable to spell orally.
Written Expression	**Copying:** Able to copy written words and recalls them to use communicate in telegraphic writing.
	Writing to Dictation: Unable to write numbers or letters to dictation.
	Self-generated: Able to write numbers in sequence to 20 and names of family members and close friends. Self-generated writing is only at basic, simple word
	Written Spelling: Fair to good at the word level.
	Drawing: Functional for communicating wants/needs.
Cognition	**Attention/Concentration:** Very good.
	Visuospatial Skills: WFL
	Memory: Long-term memory and working memory intact for procedural, semantic, and episodic systems.
	Executive Functions: WFL for planning activities of daily living (ADLs).
Behavioral Symptoms	**Alertness:** Alert and cooperative.
	Deficit awareness: Aware of his limitations.
	Frustration: Appropriate to social context; demonstrates anxiety as task complexity increases.
	Emotional Lability: None.
	Current Personality Characteristics: Pleasant and motivated; no change from pre-morbid state.

Figure 3–2. Diagnostic profile for Maurice.

abstract paragraph levels, in both modalities, he has more difficulty comprehending than at the simple sentence level. Based on observation and family report, Maurice demonstrates a consistent ability to attend to therapeutic tasks when visual stimuli are provided. This is a good prognosticator for Maurice's ability to participate in therapy.

Maurice's speech production capabilities are severely limited and this causes him great frustration, to the point of anger. His apraxia of speech combined with his dysarthria render most of his verbal output unintelligible, despite relatively spared prosody. Therefore, speech is not Maurice's strongest communication modality but as he has intact visual motor skills, writing can be his primary communication modality.

Maurice's visuospatial skills for drawing and writing were functional, although his written letters are larger than the norm, and there are misspellings and omissions. However, it is possible that writing can be optimized for communication purposes. Also consistent with his strong visuospatial skills, Maurice is also able to follow a geographic route, and has a good visual memory, which has functional value in public venues.

Maurice's executive functions were not significantly affected by his stroke. For example, his episodic memory for recent events in his daily life is preserved and that allows him to remain connected to those around him. Maurice is able to solve simple problems necessary to complete his activities of daily living, for example, prepare food, request refills of his medications, and judge dangerous situations in the home and in the community. Although Maurice cannot

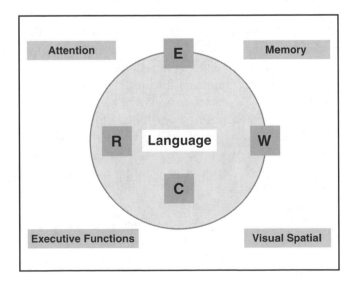

Figure 3–3. The ALD Target Model for Maurice.

communicate verbally in a functional way, his intact executive functions, functional auditory comprehension, and writing ability all serve to keep him woven into the social fabric.

Critical Thinking/Learning Activity

- What information indicates that this patient is a Broca's aphasic?
- This patient would most likely be seen in outpatient therapy. Knowing that the insurance carrier will give you a limited number of sessions, how would you prioritize this patient's functional outcomes?
- What are the family counseling and education issues in this case, and how would you address them?
- How would you include the family/caregivers in this patient's treatment plan?
- Write a SOAP note on this patient. Assume that you are seeing him for the first time after the evaluation session. Include three short-term therapeutic objectives in your note.

Treatment Considerations

Maurice was able to produce 1- to 2-syllable words that were largely unintelligible. His repetition attempts were at the 2-to-3 word phrase level. He was able to comprehend language at the phrase and sentence level and 85% at the paragraph level. Therefore, treatment for Maurice must include methods that improve his expressive output.

- Use a rhythm or melodic-based approach (MIT) to increase his MLU.
- Maurice independently began to use gestures with the nonparalyzed left-hand. The Nonsymbolic Movements for Activation of Intention (NMAI) program may optimize this functional skill.
- Encourage Maurice to use monosyllabic and bisyllabic words as opposed to polysyllabic words to minimize the effects of apraxia of speech.
- Associate a drawing to represent a particular consonant's sound. For example, "bubbles" may be drawn to represent the sound /b/; a "snake" to represent the sound /s/, etc. Then blending these sounds together with a vowel to form a CVC syllable may facilitate coarticulation. This has the potential of minimizing the effects of the apraxia of speech.
- Develop an alternative communication system for Maurice in the form of a picture book to augment verbal communication. This book should include pictorial representations of family members, friends, and activities of daily living (ADL).

Some Therapeutic Options

- Melodic Intonation Therapy (MIT) (Sparks, Helm, & Albert, 1974; Sparks & Holland, 1976).
- Nonsymbolic Movements for Activation of Intention (NMAI) (Richards, Singletary, Gonzalez Rothi, & Shirley Koehler, 2002).
- Stimulation-Facilitation Approach (Schuell, Jenkins, & Jiménez-Pabón, 1964).
- Speech Production Program for Aphasia (SPPA) (Helms-Estabrooks & Nicholas, 2000).
- Promoting Aphasics' Communicative Effectiveness (PACE) (Davis & Wilcox, 1981).
- Visual Action Therapy (VAT) (Helm-Estabrooks, Fitzpatrick, & Barresi, 1982).
- Response Elaboration Training (RET) (Kearns, 1985).
- MossTalk (Fink, Brecher, Montgomery, & Schwartz, 2003).

References

Basso, A. (2003). *Aphasia and its therapy*. New York: Oxford University Press.

Davis, G. A. (2007). *Aphasiology: Disorders and clinical practice* (2nd ed.). Boston: Pearson.

Davis, G. A., & Wilcox, M. J. (1981). Incorporating parameters of natural conversation in aphasia treatment. In R. Chapey (Ed.), *Language intervention strategies in adult aphasia.* Baltimore: Williams & Wilkins.

Fink, R., Brecher, A., Montgomery, M., & Schwartz, M. (2003). *MossTalk*. Philadelphia: Albert Einstein Healthcare Network.

Helm-Estabrooks, N., Fitzpatrick, P. M., & Barresi, B. (1982). Visual action therapy for global aphasia. *Journal of Speech and Hearing Disorders, 47,* 385–389.

Helm-Estabrooks, N., & Nicholas, M. (2000). *Sentence production program for aphasia* (2nd ed.). Austin, TX: Pro-Ed.

Johnson, A. F., & Jacobson, B. H. (2007). *Medical speech-language pathology: A practitioner's guide.* New York: Thieme.

Kearns, K. (1985). Response elaboration training for patient-initiated utterances. In R. Brookshire (Ed.), *Clinical aphasiology conference proceedings* (pp. 196–204). Minneapolis, MN: BRK.

LaPointe, L. (2005). *Aphasia and related neurogenic language disorders* (3rd ed.). New York: Thieme.

Richards, K., Singletary., F., Gonzalez-Rothi, L. J., & Koehler, S. (2002). Activation of intentional mechanism through utilization of nonsymbolic movements in aphasia rehabilitation. *Journal of Rehabilitation Research and Development, 39,* 445–454.

Rosenbek, J. C., Kent, D. R., & LaPointe, L. L. (1989). Apraxia of speech: An overview and some perspectives. In J. C. Rosenbek, M. R. McNeil, & A. E. Aronson (Eds.), *Apraxia of speech* (pp. 1–28). San Diego, CA: College-Hill Press.

Schuell, H., Jenkins, J. H., & Jiménez-Pabón, E. (1965). *Aphasia in adults: Diagnosis, prognosis and treatment.* New York: Harper & Row.

Sparks, R., Helm, N., & Albert, M. (1974). Aphasia rehabilitation resulting from melodic intonation therapy. *Cortex, 10,* 303–316.

Sparks, R., & Holland, A. (1976). Method: Melodic intonation therapy. *Journal of Speech and Hearing Disorders, 41,* 287–297.

Thompson, C. K. (2008). Treatment of syntactic and morphologic deficits in agrammatic aphasia: Treatment of the underlying forms. In R. Chapey (Ed.), *Language intervention strategies in aphasia and related neurogenic communication disorders* (5th ed., pp. 735–755). Philadelphia: Wolters Kluwer/Lippincott Williams & Wilkins.

Transcortical Motor Aphasia

Characteristics

Lichtheim (1895) referred to the aphasic disturbances due to lesions outside of the area around the sylvian fissure as *transcortical aphasias*. Transcortical motor aphasia (TMA) is a nonfluent type of aphasia. One of the distinguishing features of the transcortical aphasias, motor and sensory (which will be discussed separately), is that repetition is preserved. (Webb & Adler, 2008). More often, lesions are subcortical and located anterior to the frontal horn of the left lateral ventricle, part of the anterior watershed area, which prompted Benson (1979) to name them *border zone aphasias*. Other areas implicated in TMA involve the prefrontal and premotor cortices (Damasio, 2008). The lesions causing TMA are smaller than those causing Broca's aphasia although there may be damage to the white matter below Broca's area. It is also possible that this type of lesion may interrupt communication between Broca's region and the basal ganglia and/or the thalamus, since there are areas in these regions that may have premotor capabilities. The prognosis for a person with TMA is good due to the spared linguistic features of this disorder (Alexander & Schmitt, 1980). Typically, progress occurs early after onset.

There are three primary patterns typically seen with TMA:

1. Frontal lobe lesion affecting middle cerebral artery area (MCA) = motor speech deficits
2. Frontal lobe lesion affecting anterior cerebral artery area (ACA) = lack of spontaneous speech
3. Lesion in watershed area between MCA and ACA typically due to vascular pathology (most common)

Besides stroke, the clinician may also see frontal lobe pathology in individuals who have suffered trauma, tumor, and other progressive neuropathologies (Cimino-Knight, Hollingsworth, & Gonzales-Rothi (2005). Therefore, having a clear understanding of the relationship between lesion site and linguistic function is always very helpful when confronted with these "border zone" disturbances.

The person with TMA manifests communication difficulties which are most obvious at the conversational level. These patients initially may present as mute due to the absence of the impulse to speak. When they do initiate, they produce syntactically correct utterances, but overall they have significantly reduced verbal output. This forces their communication partner to carry the burden of the communicative event. Their best performance is noted in short, highly structured communication scenarios, as opposed to situations characterized by many open-ended questions and free-flowing exchanges. They do best when the exchange requires few words of high predictability. For example, a person with TMA would struggle to answer the question, "What brought you to the hospital?" whereas a question such as, "How many children do you have?" would be more easily answered. The information below is from Goodglass and Kaplan (1982) and describes the common features of transcortical motor aphasia:

- Nonfluent language
- Repetition is intact compared to limited speech output
- Paraphasia is evident, especially phonemic type
- Syntax errors
- Perseveration
- Difficulty initiating conversation
- Difficulty organizing responses in conversation
- Syntactic errors
- Confrontation naming is preserved.
- Auditory comprehension is excellent.
- Articulation is fair to good, though rate may be slow.
- Repetition is normal.

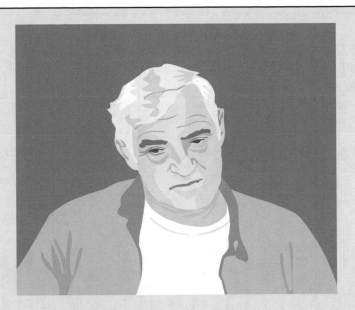

Case Scenario: Vincent

History and Physical (H & P): 75-year-old, right-handed, male Caucasian, admitted to local hospital. Right hemiparesis involving the lower extremity only was evident. On examination, he ambulated well. Family brought him to the hospital describing him as "mute." Blood pressure in the emergency department (ED) was 210/100 and heart rate was 92. He was aware of his inability to speak evidenced by his frustration and by pointing to his mouth and shaking his head in a "no" gesture.

Past Medical History (PMH): Vincent has no prior history of stroke. His PMH includes coronary artery disease, s/p angioplasty with stents; hyperlipidemia; left total knee replacement (TKR); seasonal allergies; obstructive sleep apnea (OSA). Sleep using a Klearway oral appliance to treat the OSA.

Social History: One adult daughter lives nearby. Vincent lives alone in an apartment complex that has an elevator. He has many friends and was a very active and socially engaged man prior to this stroke. He was an educator at the university level for 30 years before retirement at age 65.

Surgical History: Uvulo-palatal-pharyngoplasy (UPP) surgery for obstructive sleep apnea 10 years PTA (prior to this admission).

A Functional Analysis of Vincent

This patient has good auditory comprehension, intact word and sentence repetition, but nonfluent speech output. This is complicated by his lack of volitional initiation of speech. In Vincent's case, treatment is geared toward increasing volitional initiation of speech with less phonemic paraphasias. Based on observation

Language Expression

- **Automatic Speech:** WFL for counting, days of the week, alphabet with a verbal prompt to facilitate initiation.
- **Repetition Ability:** WFL for words and sentences.
- **Lexical Retrieval-Naming:** Confrontation naming compromised by initiation difficulties; better with cloze procedure.
- **Conversational Ability:** Verbal output limited; syntactic complexity reduced in attempts at longer utterances.
- **Pragmatic Skills:** Understands turn-taking; maintains eye contact, uses appropriate social gestures; however, non-fluent speech limits thorough evaluation of speech acts.
- **Paraphasias:** Phonemic paraphasias.

Speech

- **Rate:** Slow and halting.
- **Intelligibility:** WFL in known and unknown contexts.
- **Prosody:** Reduced intonation contours, stress pattern altered.
- **Articulation:** WFL
- **Fluency:** Speech output is non-fluent; struggles to produce utterances in response to open-ended questions. Speech output is fluent on repetition tasks.

Auditory Comprehension

- **Answering Yes/No Questions:** WFL
- **Executing Commands:** WFL
- **Understanding Stories & Paragraphs:** WFL
- **Understanding Conversational Speech:** WFL at conversational level.
- **Identifying Objects & their Functions:** WFL

Reading

- **Word-level Comprehension:** WFL
- **Sentence-level Comprehension:** WFL at paragraph level.
- **Oral Reading:** Reading aloud is difficult to produce fluently and is slow and labored.
- **Oral Spelling:** Unable to test due to non-fluent speech.

Written Expression

- **Copying:** WFL
- **Writing to Dictation:** Unable to initiate writing to dictation secondary to an ideomotor apraxia.
- **Self-generated:** Functional for name and address, when not prompted verbally.
- **Written Spelling:** Paragraphic.
- **Drawing:** If self-initiated, he is able to produce simple line drawings.

Cognition

- **Attention/Concentration:** Attends to a task when his frustration is manageable.
- **Visuospatial Skills:** WFL
- **Memory:** Procedural memory is WFL; semantic memory for basic information is intact; episodic memory difficult to assess due to limited expression.
- **Executive Functions:** Problem solving, safety awareness, and judgment are intact for ADL needs.

Behavioral Symptoms

- **Alertness:** WFL
- **Deficit awareness:** He is aware of his communication deficits.
- **Frustration:** Demonstrates intermittent frustration with his inability to "get it out".
- **Emotional Lability:** None noted.
- **Current Personality Characteristics:** His frustration is causing anger and social isolation.

Figure 3-4. Diagnostic profile for Vincent.

and family report, Vincent's speech consists mostly of immediate imitation. Although he understands what people say to him, he is continually challenged by the frustration of not being able to respond fluently and with ease. The family may consider purchasing an augmentative-alternative communication device (AAC) for Vincent, for example, a portable computer that uses a talking software program, to supplement his verbal communication.

Cognitively, Vincent is able to attend to a task when his frustration level is manageable. His memory for information that is verbally or visually presented appears intact. Visuospatial skills remain good. This will help him negotiate his home and external environment safely. Furthermore, because of his intact visuospatial skills, Vincent can draw his messages if they have emotional valence. His problem solving skills, judgment and reasoning, and safety awareness are intact for his ADL needs. For example, Vincent can be left alone at home for a limited amount of time as he knows how to access 911 via his medical alerting system; use the phone to access family members; and prepare light meals for himself. Vincent only needs minimal assistance with his AM care due to his right lower extremity weakness.

Critical Thinking/Learning Activity

1. What features of this person's aphasia indicate that he has TMA?
2. How do you bridge the gap between immediate repetition and delayed repetition to help the patient to build longer utterances?
3. Name three activities that you could use to facilitate speech initiation. Provide a rationale for each and give a scripted example of how that would happen in the therapy room.

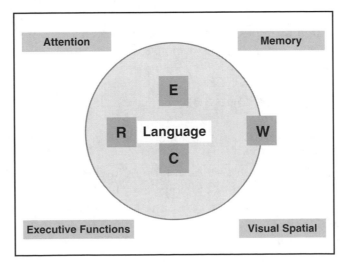

Figure 3–5. The ALD Target Model for Vincent.

4. What information would you provide to family members about TMA?
5. How would you use LPAA (life participation approach to aphasia) to facilitate functional communication in this patient?

Treatment Considerations

Vincent's treatment will focus on:

- Optimizing initiation of speech output
- Reducing paraphasic speech output
- Increasing utterance length
- Developing appropriate intonation at the sentence level

Vincent's good auditory comprehension and ability to repeat accurately could be used to support verbal output. For example, in the following task both of these preserved skills are called into play to promote speech initiation and fluency. The therapist can give Vincent a sentence supplemented with a visual stimulus (picture or object) to help him initiate and expand verbal output.

SLP: [Shows *keys* to Vincent]: I will open the door with my *keys*. What will I use to open the door? [SLP can provide a phonemic cue if needed.]

Vincent: Key.

SLP: What should I do with the key?

Vincent: Open the door.

This task allows the SLP to work not only on increasing verbal initiation and fluency, but can also help with intonation. For example, the SLP can ask, "*Who will open the door?*"

- This question prompts Vincent to respond with lexical stress on the subject of the sentence in his response.

Some Therapeutic Options

- Melodic Intonation Therapy (MIT) (Sparks, Helm, & Albert, 1974; Sparks & Holland, 1976).
- Nonsymbolic Movements for Activation of Intention (NMAI) (Richards, Singletary, Gonzalez-Rothi, & Koehler, 2002).
- Sentence Production Program for Aphasia (SPPA) (Helms-Estabrooks & Nicholas, 2000).
- Life participation approach to aphasia (LPAA) (Chapey, Duchan, Elman, Garcia, Kagan, Lyon, & Simmons-Mackie, 2008).

References

Alexander, M. P., & Schmitt, M. A. (1980). The aphasia syndrome of stroke in the left anterior cerebral artery territory. *Archives of Neurology, 37,* 97–100.

Chapey, R., Duchan, J. F., Elman, R. J., Garcia, L. J., Kagan, A., Lyon, J., et al. (2008). Life-participation approach to aphasia: A statement of values for the future. In R. Chapey (Ed.), *Language intervention strategies in aphasia and related neurogenic communication disorders* (5th ed., pp. 403–449). Philadelphia: Wolters Kluwer/Lippincott Williams & Wilkins.

Cimino-Knight, A. M., Hollingsworth, A. L., & Gonzales-Rothi, L. J. (2005). The transcortical aphasias. In L. L. LaPointe (Ed.), *Aphasia and related neurogenic language disorders* (3rd ed., pp. 169–185). New York: Thieme.

Damasio, H. (2008). Neural basis of language disorders. In R. Chapey (Ed.), *Language intervention strategies in aphasia and related neurogenic communication disorders* (5th ed., pp. 20–41). Philadelphia: Wolters Kluwer/Lippincott Williams & Wilkins.

Goodglass, H., & Kaplan, E. (1982). *The assessment of aphasia and related disorders.* Philadelphia: Lea & Febiger.

Helm-Estabrooks, N., & Nicholas, M. (2000). *Sentence production program for aphasia* (2nd ed.). Austin, TX: Pro-Ed.

Lichtheim, L. (1895). On aphasia. *Brain, 7,* 433–484.

Richards, K., Singletary., F., Gonzalez-Rothi, L. J., & Koehler, S. (2002). Activation of intentional mechanism through utilization of nonsymbolic movements in aphasia rehabilitation. *Journal of Rehabilitation Research and Development, 39,* 445–454.

Sparks, R., Helm, N., & Albert, M. (1974). Aphasia rehabilitation resulting from melodic intonation therapy. *Cortex, 10,* 303–316.

Sparks, R., & Holland, A. (1976). Method: Melodic intonation therapy. *Journal of Speech and Hearing Disorders, 41,* 287–297.

Webb, W. G., & Adler, R. K. (2008). *Neurology for the speech-language pathologist.* St. Louis, MO: Mosby Elsevier.

Global Aphasia

Characteristics

Global aphasia is a severe impairment of communication that involves all language modalities. Milder forms of global aphasia are often referred to as mixed aphasia. The incidence of global aphasia is noted to be as high as 10 to 40% of all strokes (Peach, 2001). The pathophysiology of global aphasia is a large perisylvian lesion typically greater than 6 cm. It involves damage to the frontal, temporal, and parietal lobes.

The pathophysiology is especially prominent in the posterior temporal gyrus. The infarct is secondary to abnormalities in both branches of the middle cerebral artery (MCA). This lesion also extends deep into the subadjacent white matter. Certain focal lesions within this damaged area can degrade the white matter and result in a disconnection between interacting brain regions. Possible sequellae to this disconnection are behavioral dysfunctions. According to Basso and Farabola (1997), the pathophysiology of the stroke has a bearing on the prognosis in global aphasia (Figure 3–6).

Auditory comprehension will improve more than verbal expression. Patients with global aphasia make the most gains during the first six months of recovery (Collins, 2005). However, prognosis for recovery is poor, dependent on lesion site, as noted in Figure 3–6. Also, prognosis in global aphasia is affected by the size of the lesion, that is, the larger the infracted area, the worse the prognosis. Sometimes the globally aphasic individual will not have an accompanying hemiparesis. If motor abilities are preserved the prognosis for recovery is better. If auditory comprehension and verbal expression are both severely impaired, then prognosis for recovery is poorer. Of particular importance is the patient's ability to successfully answer simple yes/no questions. The higher the accuracy of such responses, the better the prognosis for recovery.

The most salient characteristic of global aphasia is that the patient is impaired in all areas of language competence. They will present with deficits in comprehension and expression for syntax, semantics, and phonology. It is inconclusive whether the deficits in verbal expression are due to a lack of knowledge for linguistic rules and operations, that is, *linguistic competence*; or due instead to an individual's language competence *and* performance deficits (Peach, 2008). The auditory comprehension skills of individuals with global aphasia are variable. Research shows that the individual's auditory comprehension skills likely to be preserved are familiar environmental

Type	Lesion	Outcome
I.	Large Pre-and Post-Rolandic middle cerebral artery infarcts	Very poor prognosis
II.	Pre-Rolandic	Prognosis good for recovery
III.	Subcortical	Prognosis good for recovery
IV.	Parietal	Variable; improving to Broca's or Transcortical Aphasia
V.	Double frontal and Parietal	Variable; improving to Broca's or Transcortical Aphasia

Figure 3–6. Lesion type and outcome in global aphasia.

sounds, for example, a toilet flushing, a car horn, a siren, etc. (Spinnler & Vignolo, 1966); names of famous people (Van Lancker & Klein, 1990); auditory recognition of word categories, for example, food, clothing (McKenna & Warrington, 1978); and better comprehension for personally relevant information (Wallace & Stapleton, 1991). In the acute phase, the individual who performs better on auditory comprehension measures has a more favorable prognosis.

It is important to understand that persons with global aphasia are not mute. They have the ability to verbalize despite the extensive lesion, but utterances tend to be stereotypic, and they are unable to repeat. One utterance may be the extent of this person's speech output, for example, "Oh boy." This type of patient may also only produce neologistic speech, for example, "pifa, pifa." Interestingly, although prosody may be within normal limits in this patient population, it has no communicative intent and

therefore the utterance is meaningless (de Bleser & Poeck, 1985). This patient population relies most heavily on nonverbal communication for understanding the message, for example, tone of voice, facial expression, and gestures (Herrmann et al., 1989).

Cognitively, the individual with global aphasia may demonstrate problems with abstract reasoning. Research has shown that there is a correlation between language ability and abstract reasoning in the globally aphasic patient. For example, nonverbal performance on the Raven's Colored Progressive Matrices (Raven, 1965) is impaired in this patient population (Collins, 1986). This test requires that the patient complete a sequence of geometric shapes and colors. People with Wernicke's aphasia and globally aphasic patients both scored equally low compared to other types of aphasic patients on pattern completion. It appears that the more posterior the lesion, the more this type of cognition is affected.

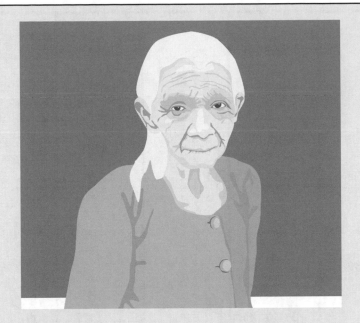

Case Scenario: Elizabeth

History and Physical (H & P): 85-year-old female, right-handed, admitted via ED with change in mental status. A CT scan revealed a massive left-sided CVA with right-sided hemiparesis and oral pharyngeal dysphagia.

Past Medical History (PMH): Gastrointestinal bleed, atrial fibrillation (A-fib), anemia, hypertension (HTN), irritable bowel syndrome (IBS), mitral valve regurgitation (MVR), history of gastric ulcers, and severe macular degeneration.

Social History: Widowed, four children, worked as a librarian; lives alone in first floor apartment in a senior citizens complex.

Surgical History: Left total knee replacement (left TKR)

A Functional Case Analysis for Elizabeth

Elizabeth has severe deficits in expressive language output. Her utterances are meaningless and lack grammatical form. Furthermore, her ability to use the verbal modality is compromised by her apraxia of speech. Elizabeth relies on reading facial expressions and gestures in order to comprehend a message so her therapist can use this as a foundation for rehabilitation. In addition, Elizabeth may be a candidate for an augmentative communication system (Steele, 2006) because she can match words and pictures with fairly consistent accuracy. Elizabeth's auditory comprehension requires intervention so that she can answer yes/no questions and follow basic directions with more reliability. This is crucial for the completion of her ADLs. Even with a home health aide present, Elizabeth still needs to be able to respond to concrete questions relating to her health and basic wants

Language Expression
- **Automatic Speech:** None.
- **Repetition Ability:** None.
- **Lexical Retrieval-Naming:** None.
- **Conversational Ability:** No connected discourse and occasional meaningless utterances.
- **Pragmatic Skills:** Cannot validly assess.
- **Paraphasias:** Undetermined due to lack of intelligible output.

Speech
- **Rate:** Non-verbal.
- **Intelligibility:** Cannot assess secondary to non-verbal status.
- **Prosody:** Cannot assess secondary to non-verbal status.
- **Articulation:** Cannot assess secondary to non-verbal status.
- **Fluency:** Absent.

Auditory Comprehension
- **Answering Yes/No Questions:** Mildly impaired for concrete/personal yes/no questions.
- **Executing Commands:** Mildly impaired accuracy for simple commands.
- **Understanding Stories & Paragraphs:** Poor.
- **Understanding Conversational Speech:** Poor.
- **Identifying Objects & their Functions:** Mildly impaired but better with real objects.

Reading
- **Word-level Comprehension:** Moderate-severely impaired for sentences; better at CVC word level.
- **Sentence-level Comprehension:** Poor.
- **Oral Reading:** Unable to assess decoding skills due to unintelligible speech output.
- **Oral Spelling:** Unable to assess oral spelling skills due to unintelligible speech output.

Written Expression
- **Copying:** Able to copy simple forms with the left hand.
- **Writing to Dictation:** Could not form letters or numbers.
- **Self-generated:** Attempts made, but unable to complete a word.
- **Written Spelling:** Could not form letters or numbers.
- **Drawing:** Can generate gross shapes but detailed features are missing.

Cognition
- **Attention/Concentration:** Limited and requires tactile cues.
- **Visuospatial Skills:** Impaired for detailed drawing and personal navigation within a building.
- **Memory:** Functional for procedural memory.
- **Executive Functions:** Unable to determine due to receptive and expressive language impairments.

Behavioral Symptoms
- **Alertness:** Variable; optimal in the morning hours.
- **Deficit awareness:** Demonstrates variable levels of awareness.
- **Frustration:** Frustrated when stimuli becomes too complex.
- **Emotional Lability:** Patient's crying is likely due to frustration and not lability.
- **Current Personality Characteristics:** Depressed and anxious.

Figure 3–7. Diagnostic profile for Elizabeth.

and needs. Cognitively, she appears to be able to attend during certain times of the day, more often in the morning hours. Her memory for family members, her biographical past, and rituals of self-care appear intact. Due to her limited executive functioning and severe language disorder, Elizabeth requires maximum supervision in the home environment. Consequently, home care services for speech and language and other areas of need should be considered, as her social communication, communication of basic needs, and daily planning need to be addressed.

Critical Thinking/Learning Activity

- What information indicates that this patient has global aphasia?
- This patient would most likely be seen in outpatient therapy. Knowing that the insurance carrier will give you a limited number of sessions, how would you prioritize this patient's therapy goals to achieve long-term functional outcomes?
- What are the family counseling and education issues in this case, and how would you address them?
- How would you include the family/caregivers in this patient's treatment plan?
- Write a SOAP note on this patient. Assume that you are seeing her for the first time after the evaluation session. Include short-term therapeutic objectives in your note.
- What aspect of this patient's medical history made this patient susceptible to stroke?

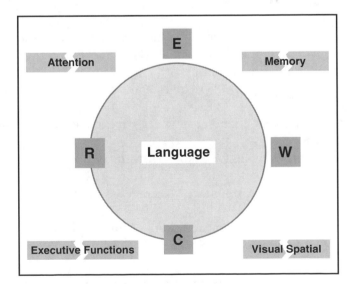

Figure 3–8. The ALD Target Model for Elizabeth.

Treatment Considerations

Elizabeth is severely impaired in language, both receptively and expressively. She does not display any functional speech. She has severe buccofacial apraxia and apraxia of speech, further complicating her functional communication abilities. Therefore, speech production is not considered a viable mode of communication at this time. Answering yes/no questions is easier for Elizabeth when they pertain to emotionally charged information, family members, recent events, and her illness. Elizabeth can recognize objects and has some residual reading comprehension for basic words when printed in large letters with accompanying realistic pictures. She can identify one of three pictured items. She can copy simple line drawings.

- To improve ability to make her needs known, a computer-based program (Steele, 2006) may be beneficial. This speech-generating device provides large icons for vocabulary that speak in a human voice. This may be used to obtain basic core vocabulary.
- Attempt to convey messages and make needs known by generating simple line drawings.
- Attempt to build upon her ability to make simple line drawings as a form of communication.
- Use a trace and copy word recall strategy.
- Elizabeth attempts to understand speech by watching facial expressions and gestures. Therefore, optimize auditory comprehension by using facial expressions, voice, gesture, and pictures to follow basic, one-step directions.

Some Therapeutic Options

- AAC (Augmentative Alternative Communication) systems should be considered, for example, from simple communication boards to more complex word-picture systems.
- Visual Action Therapy (VAT) (Helm-Estabrooks, Fitzpatrick, & Barresi, 1982).
- Promoting Aphasics Communication Effectiveness (PACE) (Davis & Wilcox, 1985).
- Communicative Drawing Program (CDP) (Helm-Estabrooks & Albert, (2004).
- Voluntary Control of Involuntary Utterances (VCIU) (Helm & Barresi, 1980).
- Nonsymbolic Movements for Activation of Intention (NMAI) (Richards, Singletary, Gonzalez-Rothi, & Koehler, 2002).

References

Basso, A., & Farabola, M. (1997). Comparison of improvement of pahsia in three patients with lesions in anterior, posterior, and antero-posterior language areas. *Neuropsychological Rehabilitation*, 7, 215–230.

Collins, M. (1986). *Diagnosis and treatment of global aphasia.* San Diego, CA: College-Hill Press.

Collins, M. (2004). Global aphasia. In L. LaPointe (Ed.), *Aphasia and related neurogenic language disorders* (3rd ed., pp. 186–198). New York: Thieme.

Davis, G. A., & Wilcox, M. (1985). *Adult aphasia rehabilitation: Applied pragmatics.* San Diego, CA: College-Hill Press.

de Bleser, R., & Poeck, K. (1985). Analysis of prosody in the spontaneous speech of patients with CV-recurring utterances. *Cortex*, 21, 405–416.

Helm, N. A., & Barresi, B. (1980). Voluntary control of involuntary utterances: A treatment approach for severe aphasia. *Clinical Aphasiology*, 10, 308–315.

Helm-Estabrooks, N., & Albert, M. L. (2004). *Manual of aphasia and aphasia therapy* (2nd ed.). Austin, TX: Pro-Ed.

Helm-Estabrooks, N., Fitzpatrick, P. M., & Barresi, B. (1982). Visual action therapy for global aphasia. *Journal of Speech and Hearing Disorders*, 47, 385–389.

Herrmann, M., Koch, U., Johannsen-Horbach, H., & Wallesch, C. W. (1989). Communicative skills in chronic and severe nonfluent aphasia. *Brain and Language*, 37, 339–352.

McKenna, P., & Warrington, E. K. (1978). Category-specific naming preservation: A single-case study. *Journal of Neurology, Neurosurgery, and Psychiatry*, 41, 571–574.

Peach, A. R. (2008). Global aphasia: Identification and management. In R. Chapey (Ed.), *Language intervention strategies in aphasia and related neurogenic communication disorders* (5th ed., pp. 565–594). Philadelphia: Wolters Kluwer/Lippincott Williams & Wilkins.

Raven, J. C. (1965). *Guide to using the colored progressive matrices.* London: H. K. Lewis.

Richards, K., Singletary, F., Gonzalez-Rothi, L. J., & Koehler, S. (2002). Activation of intentional mechanism through utilization of nonsymbolic movements in aphasia rehabilitation. *Journal of Rehabilitation Research and Development*, 39, 445–454.

Spinnler, H., & Vignolo, L. (1996). Impaired recognition of meaningful sounds in aphasia. *Cortex*, 2, 337–348.

Steele, R. D. (2006). AAC use and communicative improvements in chronic aphasia: Evidence comparing global with severe Broca's aphasia. *AAC Perspectives (ASHA SID-12)*, 15(4), 18–22.

Van Lancker, D., & Klein, K. (1990). Preserved recognition of familiar personal names in global aphasia. *Brain and Language*, 39, 511–529.

Wallace, G. L., & Stapleton, J. H. (1991). Analysis of auditory comprehension performance in individuals with severe aphasia. *Archives of Physical Medicine and Rehabilitation*, 72, 674–678.

Chapter 4

THE MAJOR FLUENT APHASIC SYNDROMES

Wernicke's Aphasia

Characteristics

Carl Wernicke described the language disorder now bearing his name in 1908. Wernicke's aphasia is also referred to as *receptive aphasia*, *sensory aphasia*, and *posterior aphasia*. The lesion producing Wernicke's aphasia is at the anatomic intersection for all incoming auditory and visual information (Figure 4–1). Wernicke's aphasia results from a lesion in the posterior third of the superior temporal gyrus. Blood supply to this area is via the inferior division of the middle cerebral artery (MCA). Therefore, reading, writing, repetition, and other language functions are often impaired (Marshall, 2001, p. 435). Primarily temporal lesions produce word deafness and reading is less affected. In this variant, auditory comprehension for words in context is better than words in isolation. The second variant of this type of aphasia results from a more posterior lesion of the temporal gyrus, which affects the visual connections. Consequently, reading comprehension is impaired in this patient population. Oral reading tends to be intact, but reading comprehension is affected. Those affected will have difficulty recognizing letters by name, and difficultly associating written words with their spoken counterparts. Writing is characterized by paragraphic jargon, similar to speech. Spelling is severely impaired. These individuals are better able to understand words in isolation as opposed to words in context, unlike the patients with the more anterior lesion.

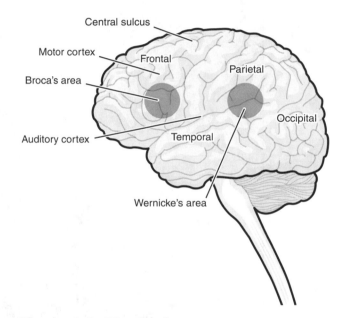

Figure 4–1. Wernicke's area.

A hallmark of Wernicke's aphasia is a significant auditory comprehension problem with poor self-monitoring. Paraphasic speech is common and typically goes unnoticed by the speaker. The speech is effortless and melodic; however, there are verbal (semantic) and literal (phonemic) paraphasias and in more severe cases neologisms are used, all of which go unnoticed due to poor self-monitoring skills. As a result, the person with Wernicke's aphasia has speech output with very low informational content. Articulation is unimpaired; however, they have poorly chosen words and poorly formed sentences, which tend to be paragrammatic, that is, they omit grammatical morphemes. Their self-initiated output tends to be more contextually appropriate than communication in dyadic discourse. This is due to their problems in the comprehension of the communicative partner's speech. The patient may also demonstrate a press for speech, or logorrhea. Interestingly, hemiparesis is not common in this patient population as the lesion is posterior to motor functions mediated in the frontal lobes. In comparison to the other fluent aphasias, Wernicke's is the most severe and has the poorest prognosis. LaPointe (1997) reports that one marker of their prognosis for recovery is based on their auditory comprehension for single words.

These patients can also demonstrate paranoid tendencies in addition to a general lack of awareness of their language difficulties. They can be resistant to therapy since they do not understand its value. Therefore, two primary goals with these patients are to improve auditory comprehension and self-monitoring of errors (Brookshire, 1997).

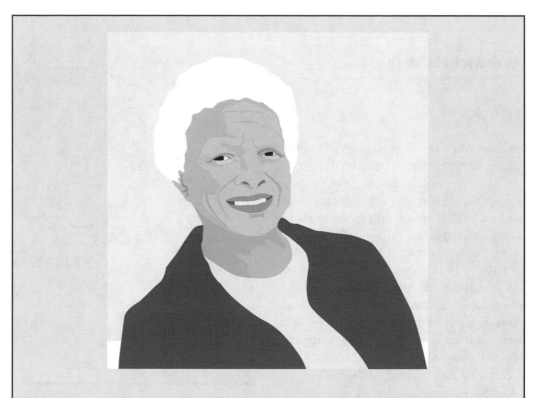

Case Scenario: Mildred

History and Physical (H & P): 68-year-old female, right-handed, found down by neighbor who called 911; alert but aphasic in ED; preliminary CT scan revealed a CVA in the middle cerebral artery (MCA) distribution territory posterior to the central sulcus and superior to the sylvian fissure. There was no observable hemiparesis.

Past Medical History (PMH): Insulin Dependent Diabetes Mellitus (IDDM); hypertension; hyperlipidemia; A-fib; COPD; depression.

Social History: Widowed, lives alone; sedentary lifestyle; no family in area.

Surgical History: Cholecystectomy, appendectomy; hysterectomy.

Language Expression

- **Automatic Speech:** Poor. Paraphasias noted in a counting sequence from 1–20; perseveration noted after the number 5.
- **Repetition Ability:** Poor for words and sentences.
- **Lexical Retrieval-Naming:** Circumlocutions and semantic paraphasias and neologisms noted on confrontation naming tasks.
- **Conversational Ability:** Devoid of content; press of speech with numerous paraphasias and neologisms; paragrammatic with omissions of tense markers, prefixes, etc.
- **Pragmatic Skills:** Poor awareness of turn-taking rules; inappropriate social language.
- **Paraphasias:** Frequent semantic, phonemic paraphasias and neologisms.

Speech

- **Rate:** WFL
- **Intelligibility:** WFL in all contexts.
- **Prosody:** Normal intonation patterns noted.
- **Articulation:** WFL
- **Fluency:** Logorrheic but devoid of content; "press of speech" noted; numerous paraphasias.

Auditory Comprehension

- **Answering Yes/No Questions:** Moderate ability to answer concrete questions and significant difficulty with abstract yes/no questions. Echolalia is present.
- **Executing Commands:** Moderate impairment at the simple one-step level.
- **Understanding Stories & Paragraphs:** Severely impaired.
- **Understanding Conversational Speech:** Severely impaired with an inability to self-monitor for errors.
- **Identifying Objects & their Functions:** Moderately impaired when asked to point an object from a field of three.

Reading

- **Word-level Comprehension:** Severe alexia; sound-symbol disassociation; unable to read at the word level.
- **Sentence-level Comprehension:** Poor.
- **Oral Reading:** Difficulty associating written words with spoken counterparts and their meanings.
- **Oral Spelling:** Severely impaired.

Written Expression

- **Copying:** WFL given interest.
- **Writing to Dictation:** Breaks in the words are noted during writing to dictation.
- **Self-generated:** Writes with ease but letterforms are inconsistently correct; fluent paragraphic jargon similar to speech with no awareness of errors.
- **Written Spelling:** Severely impaired.
- **Drawing:** Functional for communicating ADL needs.

Cognition

- **Attention/Concentration:** Requires, tactile, verbal and/or visual prompts for sustained attention.
- **Visuospatial Skills:** WFL for ADL needs.
- **Memory:** Procedural memory appears intact for ADL needs; visual memory is a strength; semantic and episodic memory difficult to assess due to comprehension deficits.
- **Executive Functions:** Problem solving/judgment for safety purposes intact.

Behavioral Symptoms

- **Alertness:** More alert in the AM hours and when frustration is low.
- **Deficit awareness:** No awareness of deficits (anosagnosia); poor self-monitoring of output.
- **Frustration:** More frustrated with others causing anger and lashing out verbally.
- **Emotional Lability:** None.
- **Current Personality Characteristics:** Depressed, anxious, angry, and tense which is dissimilar to her pre-morbid state.

Figure 4–2. Diagnostic profile for Mildred.

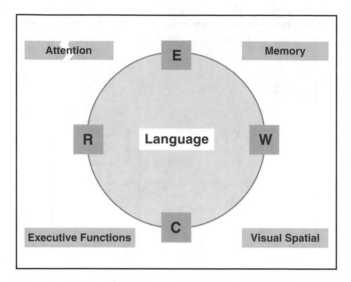

Figure 4–3. ALD Target Model for Mildred.

A Functional Analysis of Mildred's Wernicke's Aphasia

Mildred's receptive language skills are the most impaired. Consequently, she is unable to participate as a conversational partner for two primary reasons: (1) her logorrhea is unchecked due to her inability to self-monitor; and (2) her output is devoid of content. Therefore, her functional expressive abilities are limited. Mildred is unable to spell so writing to communicate her needs is not possible. However, she has adequate graphomotor skills and visual perceptual skills for gross drawings, usable for communication purposes.

Cognitively, Mildred is able to attend to a task if it interests her and does not frustrate her. However, she may require tactile, verbal, and/or visual prompts for sustained attention. She wants to successfully convey messages and resorts to drawing, if prompted, when her communication partner conveys a lack of comprehension. Mildred's auditory-verbal memory span is reduced; however, visual memory is strength. Mildred is able to solve problems through action, not verbally (i.e., she can demonstrate a solution but is unable to convey it verbally due to her severely paraphasic output). For example, Mildred is able to recognize that a spilled liquid on the floor is to be avoided, so she walks around it. However, when she is asked to explain the solution, she points to the spill and says, "No, no, no watch out!" Her visuospatial skills for her gross drawings are functional, again, making this her strongest communication modality. An example of this is observed when Mildred wants something to drink and draws a crude representation of a cup while simultaneously saying, "It's a, I want it, it's a time, I want it a picka micka."

Critical Thinking/Learning Activity

■ What information indicates that this is a person with Wernicke's aphasia?

■ How would this patient's *press for speech* impact her communicative effectiveness?

■ What are the family counseling and education issues in this case, and how would you address them?

■ What are the pros and cons of encouraging the use of an AAC device in this case?

■ Write a SOAP note on this patient. Assume that you are seeing her for the first time after the evaluation session. Include three short-term therapeutic objectives in your note.

■ Discuss the impact of this patient's depression on her outcome for functional communication.

Treatment Considerations

The most important aspects of Mildred's treatment plan will include those that:

■ Optimize her auditory comprehension so that she can participate, at the most basic level, in the social context around her.

■ Give her a functional and efficacious means to communicate her wants and needs.

■ Develop the strengths that she does have to facilitate both the receptive and expressive goals mentioned above.

Some general therapeutic objectives and techniques applicable to Mildred's profile include:

■ Establish her ability to execute simple one step commands by pairing speech with gestures and picture cues to augment understanding. This may help her caregivers in better meeting her ADL needs.

■ Improve her ability to respond to simple, concrete, and personal "yes/no" questions to help her caregivers provide for her basic needs.

■ Train Mildred in recognizing the "STOP" hand gesture to facilitate a decrease in her press of speech. Consequently, she may be able to process more effectively.

■ Optimize and facilitate Mildred's drawing skills so that she can supplement her verbal output with pictorial representations of her message. This can reduce her frustration and anxiety around the issue of not being understood by her communication partner.

Some Therapeutic Options

- PACE (Promoting Aphasics' Communicative Effectiveness) (Edelman, 1987).
- Schuell's Stimulation Facilitation Approach (Coelho, Sinotte, & Duffy, 2008).
- LPAA (Life Participation Approach to Aphasia) (Chapey, Duchan, Elman, Garcia, Kagan, Lyon, & Simmons-Mackie, 2008).
- ACRT (Anagram, Copy, and Recall Treatment) (Helm-Estabrooks & Albert, 2004).

References

Brookshire, R. H. (1997). *Introduction to neurogenic communication disorders*. New York: Mosby.

Chapey, R., Duchan, J. F., Elman, R. J., Garcia, L. J., Kagan, A., Lyon, J. G., et al. (2008) Life-participation approach to aphasia: A statement of values for the future. In R. Chapey (Ed.), *Language intervention strategies in aphasia and related neurogenic communication disorders* (5th ed., pp. 279–289). Philadelphia: Wolters Kluwer/Lippincott Williams & Wilkins.

Coelho, C. A., Sinotte, M. P., & Duffy, J. R. (2008) Schuell's stimulation approach to rehabilitation. In R. Chapey (Ed.), *Language intervention strategies in aphasia and related neurogenic communication disorders* (5th ed., pp. 403–449). Philadelphia: Wolters Kluwer/Lippincott Williams & Wilkins.

Edelman, G. (1987). *P.A.C.E.: Promoting aphasics' communicative effectiveness*. Bicester, England: Winslow Press.

Helm-Estabrooks, N., & Albert, M. L. (2004). *Anagram, copy, and recall therapy. Manual of aphasia and aphasia therapy* (2nd ed). Austin, TX: Pro-Ed.

LaPointe, L. L. (1997). *Aphasia and related neurogenic language disorders* (2nd ed.). New York: Thieme.

Marshall, R. C. (2001). Early management of Wernicke's aphasia: A context-based approach. In R. Chapey (Ed.), *Language intervention strategies in aphasia and related neurogenic communication disorders* (4th ed., pp. 507–530). Philadelphia: Lippincott Williams & Wilkins.

Transcortical Sensory Aphasia

Characteristics

Transcortical Sensory Aphasia (TSA) is a rare form of fluent aphasia and the patient typically has a poor sense of the extent of their impairment. There is limited research about this form of aphasia in the rehabilitation literature. It is believed to result from vascular insufficiency in the MCA (middle cerebral artery) watershed area, that is, at the ends of the cerebral arteries. Wernicke's and Broca's areas remain intact and the arcuate fasciculus also remains undamaged but the tissue surrounding them is infarcted.

Transcortical sensory aphasia is characterized by fluent, well-articulated speech, with frequent neologisms and paraphasias, and discourse tends to be incoherent with numerous circumlocutions. People with TSA have a more favorable communication prognosis than those with Wernicke's aphasia which has a similar language profile. Individuals with TSA can repeat what is said to them by relying on the phonological system. For example, in these patients, their performance improves on verbal repetition tasks because the arcuate fasiculus remains intact. Auditory comprehension deficits vary in magnitude, although most patients have severely limited comprehension of language. Echolalia is often noted and may deceive the listener into believing that the patient is responding somewhat appropriately. Word finding difficulties are common and these patients tend to use many ready-made expressions, such as, "OK," "Ya know," "Oh, boy!" and so forth. Confrontation naming is often impaired with the patient giving meaningless responses (Goodglass & Kaplan, 2001). In summary, the most salient characteristics of TSA are intact repetition with limited comprehension and reduced propositional speech.

Interestingly, patients with early Alzheimer's dementia may present with similar symptoms to transcortical sensory aphasia and patients with vascular lesions of the left thalamic nuclei also present with TSA (Crosson, 1992). This indicates that the neuroanatomical substrate for this disorder is variable. Semantic dysfunction is often a concomitant feature due to impairment in the ability to activate the semantic system for word output. Therefore, the individual may have difficulty understanding the meaning of the word. Left posterior temporal-parietal-occipital and thalamic areas are important for vocabulary knowledge in the semantic system and these areas may be damaged in individuals with TSA. Consequently, coherent discourse and effective propositional speech are compromised.

In the TSA patient, repetition for words is usually easier than it is for sentences. Any therapeutic approach to improve verbal output should utilize common words rather than abstract words and concepts. The person with TSA often can repeat words but cannot name objects when they are seen or felt. They also have difficulty pointing to objects that are named for them. The person with TSA preserves the ability to translate a spoken sound to a written letter. This is helpful because it permits them to communicate via writing although spelling errors are noted. These errors are characterized by the regularization of irregularly spelled words, that is, the patient may write the word ignoring spelling rules. For example, "face" may be written as "fas."

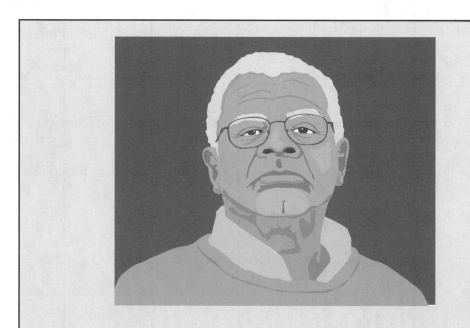

Case Scenario: John

History and Physical (H & P): 75-year-old, right-handed, African-American male, admitted to local psychiatric hospital. Hemiparesis was evident and the family noted that he had some sensory changes on the right side. On examination, he

Language Expression

Automatic Speech:	WFL for counting, days of the week, alphabet. Able to repeat lengthy prayers and lyrics.
Repetition Ability:	WFL at word and phrase levels however difficulty with longer sentences and abstract concepts.
Lexical Retrieval-Naming:	Confrontation naming is poor. Uses stereotypical phrases (i.e., "that a boy") and nonspecific words (i.e., "uh, um") as fillers and substitutions.
Conversational Ability:	Mild echolalia present in attempt to answer questions; running speech can be empty of meaning in long monologues. Syntax WFL.
Pragmatic Skills:	Turn-taking skills are functional; topic maintenance is impaired; proxemics is WFL; eye contact WFL; initiating WFL.
Paraphasias:	Occasional neologisms, circumlocutions and paraphasias (especially semantic paraphasias) are present.

Speech

Rate:	WFL
Intelligibility:	WFL
Prosody:	Rate, rhythm, and intonation were WFL.
Articulation:	WFL
Fluency:	WFL

Auditory Comprehension

Answering Yes/No Questions:	WFL for concrete and personal yes/no questions; Poor performance noted for abstract questions.
Executing Commands:	Poor performance; however, accuracy increases with visual cues.
Understanding Stories & Paragraphs:	Poor.
Understanding Conversational Speech:	Poor comprehension skills at the discourse level.
Identifying Objects & their Functions:	Poor in a field of four or more objects.

Reading

Word-level Comprehension:	Able to match simple, regularly-spelled CVC words with pictures.
Sentence-level Comprehension:	Comprehension of written language severely impaired.
Oral Reading:	Spells aloud to facilitate oral reading at the CVC word level, with minimal success.
Oral Spelling:	Able to spell simple, CVC words aloud.

Written Expression

Copying:	WFL
Writing to Dictation:	Writing words and sentences to dictation is mildly impaired.
Self-generated:	Can write words only with occasional paraphasic errors.
Written Spelling:	Spelling is functional at the CVC level for regularly spelled words.
Drawing:	Can execute simple line drawings.

Cognition

Attention/Concentration:	Varies with time of day and medical status.
Visuospatial Skills:	Adequate for reading and writing with limited text.
Memory:	To be assessed.
Executive Functions:	To be assessed.

Behavioral Symptoms

Alertness:	Variable with more confusion noted in the evening.
Deficit awareness:	No awareness of deficits (anosagnosia).
Frustration:	Demonstrates intermittent anger and frustration, especially when others do not seem to understand him.
Emotional Lability:	None noted.
Current Personality Characteristics:	Angry, frustrated, confused about his condition.

Figure 4–4. Diagnostic profile for John.

ambulated with maximum assistance. Family brought him to the hospital with echolalia and speaking in nonsense syllables that "sounded like foreign words." Blood pressure and heart rate were within normal limits for his age. He was unaware of his speech difficulty.

Past Medical History (PMH): The family reported the possibility of vascular dementia and this was confirmed by the primary care physician via a telephone call from the ED (emergency department).

Social History: Widowed, 1 adult daughter who lives nearby. John lives alone in an apartment complex that has an elevator. He has a few close friends in the complex.

Surgical History: Hernia surgery 5 years ago for inguinal tears. Cataract surgery was recently completed successfully in his left eye. The right eye is in need of cataract surgery.

A Functional Analysis of John's Transcortical Sensory Aphasia (TSA)

John's receptive language skills are the most impaired. Notice the similarities between John's TSA and Mildred's Wernicke's aphasias in this domain. Like Mildred, John was unable to effectively participate in any conversational exchanges because he was unable to self-monitor his speech errors and produced nonmeaningful output. Unlike Mildred, John was echolalic, which further complicated conversational success.

Expressively, John demonstrated normal syntax, but because of his word retrieval problems and paraphasias, his speech was empty of meaning. However,

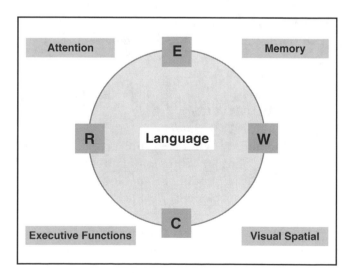

Figure 4–5. ALD Target Model for John.

his automatic speech and repetition remained largely intact and would be important to consider in treatment planning. He was unable to use writing as a communication modality. He could recognize pictures. Therefore, creating an alternative means of communication for John using a portable picture book would be an efficacious method for augmenting his communication needs. Initially, John could benefit from starting with rote, automatic information, for example, days of the week, months of the year, numbers, and so forth.

According to John's primary care physician (PCP), his vascular disease has resulted in a dementia. Therefore, further cognitive testing is indicated in this case. John's cognitive status is a critical factor in his functional success postdischarge and in outpatient therapy. If the cognitive testing demonstrates that John does have memory and executive function problems (i.e., problem-solving, reasoning, and judgment), then his ability to learn a new communication system may be compromised, especially as vascular dementia progresses. Consequently, the clinician would need to develop other treatment options in order to facilitate functional communication. Cognitive assessment, as possible, is important for the therapeutic planning and progress monitoring in the person with aphasia.

Critical Thinking/Learning Activity

- How do you intend to establish a core vocabulary with John?
- What will you use to support his acquisition and comprehension of words?
- Which of John's strengths can you use to promote use of a core vocabulary?
- How will you advance John from the word level to the sentence level, receptively and expressively?
- John produces long paraphasic utterances that compromise his intended meaning. How will you facilitate the production of short, meaningful utterances so that John can become a functional communicator of his wants and needs?
- Do you view John's echolalia as a receptive or expressive deficit? Explain.

Treatment Considerations

Persons with TSA tend to improve with repetition tasks. The list below will assist in determining how to use John's intact repetition therapeutically. Based on your findings, a treatment plan using repetition combined with another modality, at an appropriate level, may be developed.

- Compare repetition for single words versus sentences
- Compare repetition for real versus nonwords

■ Compare repetition of common versus abstract words
■ Some general therapeutic techniques applicable to John's deficit profile include:
■ Pairing auditory input with another modality, typically visual support using pictures and words.
■ Reading aloud at the word level with pictured and written support (copying may support communication as another modality).
■ Providing visual support via pictures and matching that to written and verbally presented sentences for reducing paraphasic errors.
■ Using a verbal sequencing task (picture sequence cards) to facilitate cohesive discourse.
■ Based on John's ADL needs, build a core vocabulary for improving auditory comprehension and facilitating appropriate word use in functional contexts.

Some Therapeutic Options

■ PACE (Promoting Aphasics Communicative Effectiveness) (Edelman, 1987).
■ Schuell's Stimulation Approach (Coelho, Sinotte, & Duffy, 2008).
■ Supported Conversation
■ LPAA (Life Participation Approach to Aphasia) (Chapey, Duchan, Elman, Garcia, Kagan, Lyon, & Simmons-Mackie, 2008).
■ ACRT (Anagram, Copy, and Recall Therapy) (Helm-Estabrooks & Albert, 2004).

References

Chapey, R., Duchan, J. F., Elman, R. J., Garcia, L. J., Kagan, A., Lyon, J. G., et al. (2008) Life-participation approach to aphasia: A statement of values for the future. In R. Chapey (Ed.), *Language intervention strategies in aphasia and related neurogenic communication disorders* (5th ed., pp. 279–289). Philadelphia: Wolters Kluwer/Lippincott Williams & Wilkins.

Coelho, C. A., Sinotte, M. P., & Duffy, J. R. (2008). Schuell's stimulation approach to rehabilitation. In R. Chapey (Ed.), *Language intervention strategies in aphasia and related neurogenic communication disorders* (5th ed., pp. 403–449). Philadelphia: Wolters Kluwer/Lippincott Williams & Wilkins.

Crosson, B. (1992). *Subcortical function in language and memory.* New York: Oxford University Press.

Edelman, G. (1987). *P.A.C.E.: Promoting aphasics' communicative effectiveness.* Bicester, England: Winslow Press.

Goodglass, H., & Kaplan, E. (2001). *The assessment of aphasia and related disorders.* Philadelphia: Lea & Febiger.

Helm-Estabrooks, N., & Albert, M. L. (2004). *Anagram, copy, and recall therapy. Manual of aphasia and aphasia therapy* (2nd ed). Austin, TX: Pro-Ed.

Warrington, E., & Shallice, T. (1984). Category specific semantic impairments. *Brain, 107,* 829–854.

Conduction Aphasia

Characteristics

Conduction aphasia is a fluent aphasia and can result from a lesion to the cortical region connecting Broca's and Wernicke's area. This region incorporates the supramarginal gyrus and the white matter pathways of the arcuate fasiculus as well as the superior longitudinal fasiculus. However, Broca's and Wernicke's areas remain intact. Lesion localization has been controversial regarding conduction aphasia (Geschwind, 1965). Historically, the general assumption was that a lesion to the arcuate fasiculus would result in conduction aphasia (Anderson, Gilmore, Roper, Crosson, Bauer, et al., 1999). However, Damasio (2001) indicated that the arcuate fasiculus does not need to be damaged for aphasia to be present. If the lesion is more posterior, the patient has more fluent speech.

If the lesion is more anterior and inferior, speech is less fluent and contains phonemic paraphasias.

The most salient feature of conduction aphasia is a marked difficulty with repetition, especially for function words rather than nouns, in the presence of good auditory comprehension (Chapey & Hallowell, 2001). The conduction aphasic is able to produce complex syntactic structures in spontaneous speech. However, literal (phonemic) paraphasias will interfere with effective verbal communication, despite the appropriate syntactic structures. Speech production is characterized by good intonation and fluency but due to word-finding difficulties the clinician may observe hesitations in speech output as well as circumlocutions. Reading comprehension is intact, but oral reading is characterized by literal paraphasias, omission of words and/or word substitutions. The person with conduction aphasia is able to recognize their errors and they will try to self-correct. Typically, conduction aphasia will resolve to an anomic aphasia.

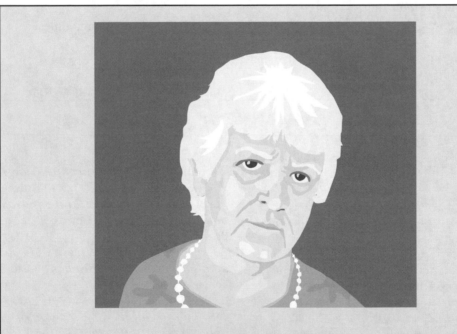

Case Scenario: Miriam

History and Physical (H & P): 67-year-old, right-handed, white female, admitted to Rehab Hospital 3 months s/p (status post) left CVA in the middle cerebral artery territory (MCA); ambulates with a straight cane, with upper and lower extremity right-sided weakness.

Language Expression

- **Automatic Speech:** WFL for counting, reciting the alphabet, stating days and months of the year.
- **Repetition Ability:** Repeating phrases moderately impaired; difficulties with multisyllabic words and with more abstract words; Spontaneous speech better than repetition. Repetition of numbers is easier than for words.
- **Lexical Retrieval-Naming:** Frequent anomia, especially on confrontation naming, with attempts to self-correct.
- **Conversational Ability:** Syntax is WFL. Ability to converse with paraphasias noted; at the conversational level, speech was circumlocutionary and paraphasic. Miriam hesitates after brief runs of fluent speech.
- **Pragmatic Skills:** WFL
- **Paraphasias:** Verbal output characterized by literal (phonemic) paraphasias.

Speech

- **Rate:** WFL
- **Intelligibility:** WFL
- **Prosody:** WFL for inflection, rhythm, and stress of speech.
- **Articulation:** WFL
- **Fluency:** Fluent; average phrase length is 7+ words. Demonstrates episodes logorrhea; tries to produce repeated approximations to self-correct speech errors. [May be mistaken for apraxia of speech]

Auditory Comprehension

- **Answering Yes/No Questions:** WFL for concrete and abstract questions.
- **Executing Commands:** WFL
- **Understanding Stories & Paragraphs:** Comprehension for sentences is intact. Difficulty with grammatical morphemes (tense, plurals).
- **Understanding Conversational Speech:** WFL; group settings pose some difficulty.
- **Identifying Objects & their Functions:** WFL

Reading

- **Word-level Comprehension:** WFL
- **Sentence-level Comprehension:** WFL
- **Oral Reading:** Minimal difficulty reading aloud at the sentence level.
- **Oral Spelling:** Paraphasic errors noted on words > 4 letters in length.

Written Expression

- **Copying:** WFL
- **Writing to Dictation:** Able to write common words to dictation.
- **Self-generated:** Writing contains spelling errors; however, words are mostly accurate in context.
- **Written Spelling:** Syllables in words are inconsistently transposed.
- **Drawing:** WFL

Cognition

- **Attention/Concentration:** WFL
- **Visuospatial Skills:** WFL
- **Memory:** Long-term memory and working memory intact for procedural, semantic, and episodic systems.
- **Executive Functions:** Planning and reasoning WFL for ADL needs.

Behavioral Symptoms

- **Alertness:** Depressed mood, however alert and cooperative for therapy.
- **Deficit awareness:** Keenly aware of speech production difficulty.
- **Frustration:** Significant frustration noted.
- **Emotional Lability:** None.
- **Current Personality Characteristics:** Depressed with feelings of hopelessness; not consistent with her premorbid personality.

Figure 4–6. Diagnostic profile for Miriam.

Past Medical History (PMH): HTN (hypertension), osteoporosis, s/p MI (myocardial infarction), h/o (history of) TIAs (transient ischemic attacks).

Social History: Married; two adult sons; husband retired policeman not supportive of patient's illness and needs; two story home, 8 steps to enter; attends an adult center during the day when at home. Patient stated that she was "depressed" over her CVA (cerebral vascular accident) and the impact it had on her ADLs (activities of daily living).

Surgical History: Unremarkable.

A Functional Analysis of Miriam's Aphasia

In general, Miriam's ability to understand conversation is good with some diminished capacity in group settings. She is able to interact appropriately with a conversational partner although she is often frustrated by her word finding difficulties. She tries repeatedly to find the correct word but this is often a struggle and she becomes angry with herself. Consequently, Miriam's verbal communication has many interruptions. Word finding and paraphasias are prevalent, making conversation challenging for both Miriam and her communication partner.

Cognitively, Miriam attends well and appears to have intact memory for information and events. She is usually correct with her answers to questions about facts and stories from the immediate and more remote past. Visuospatial skills are adequate as Miriam is able to copy and draw and she can recall print for letters and common words. Executive functioning appears within normal limits. She functions appropriately in most social settings, and is able to make her needs known. She takes care of family demands for basic cooking, light cleaning, and is planning to return to her card-game group in the community where she lives.

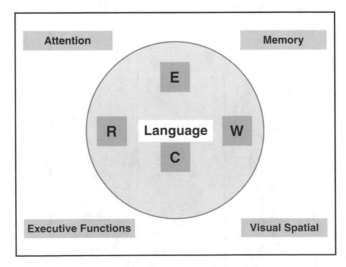

Figure 4–7. ALD Target Model for Miriam.

Critical Thinking/Learning Activity

- What characteristics of this patient's language disorder indicate that she has features of conduction aphasia?
- What are some psychosocial factors that could impact this patient's ability to effectively participate in therapy?
- What are the family counseling and educational issues in this case, and what objectives would you target?
- How would you implement an interdisciplinary plan with this patient and which other services would you include?
- Discuss an activity and materials that you believe would target several of the short-term objectives listed in the above section.

Treatment Considerations

Miriam's speech is characterized by many phonemic paraphasias; however, her prognosis for becoming a functional communicator is good. Good self-monitoring skills are an asset to her treatment although she is often frustrated by her awareness of her paraphasic speech and word finding difficulties. Repetition also presents a challenge once the words become multisyllabic, that is, greater than 3 to 4 syllables. Her good auditory comprehension and ability to write are assets to be used in program planning. Therapeutic intervention will begin where Miriam feels successful and increase in small steps, extending from concrete to more abstract stimuli. Here are some suggestions:

- Increase ability to retrieve words through: word associations, pictures, gestural cues, and sentence stem fill-ins. Avoid phonemic cues, as they are often paraphasic.
- Decrease paraphasic errors by self-monitoring and using a readily available picture-based dictionary.
- Improve repetition ability starting with easy, one-syllable words and progressing to less common multisyllabic words with written word cues, unison production, and syllable taps. However, if success is limited, consider whether repetition is a functional goal worth continuing.
- Improve sequencing of phonemes to reduce metathesis (transposing sounds and syllables within a word).
- Improve writing ability by using printed syllables on separate cards to be organized in the correct sequence and then copied.

Some Therapeutic Options

- Life Participation Approach to Aphasia (Chapey, Duchan, Elman, Garcia, Kagan, Lyon, & Simmons-Mackie, 2008).

> ■ RET (Response Elaboration Training) to improve content words used to describe a picture (Kearns & Scher, 1988).
> ■ Narrative story cards to facilitate accurate recall of information and optimize discourse skills for daily needs (Helm-Estabrooks & Nicholas, 2003).
> ■ Divergent word retrieval to stimulate word retrieval by asking the patient to visualize and name as many of a specific category (animals, food, transportation, etc.) as can be recalled (Chapey & Hallowell, 2001).

References

Anderson, J., Gilmore, R., Roper, S., Crosson, B., Bauer, R. M., Nadeau, S., et al. (1999). Conduction aphasia and the arcuate fasciculus: A reexamination of the Wernicke-Geschwind model. *Brain and Language*, *70*, 1–12.

Chapey, R., Duchan, J. F., Elman, R. J., Garcia, L. J., Kagan, A., Lyon, J. G., et al. (2008) Life-participation approach to aphasia: A statement of values for the future. In R. Chapey (Ed.), *Language intervention strategies in aphasia and related neurogenic communication disorders* (5th ed., pp. 279–289). Philadelphia: Wolters Kluwer/Lippincott Williams & Wilkins.

Chapey, R., & Hallowell, B. (2001). Introduction to language intervention strategies in adult aphasia. In R. Chapey (Ed.), *Language intervention strategies in aphasia and related neurogenic communication disorders* (4th ed., pp. 3–19). Philadelphia: Lippincott, Williams & Wilkins.

Damasio, H. (2001). Neural basis of language disorders. In R. Chapey (Ed.), *Language intervention strategies in adult aphasia and related neurogenic communication disorders* (4th ed., pp. 18–36). Philadelphia: Lippincott Williams & Wilkins.

Geschwind, N. (1965). Disconnection syndromes in animals and man. *Brain*, *88*, 237–294.

Helm-Estabrooks, N., & Nicholas, M. (2003). *Narrative story cards*. Austin, TX: Pro-Ed.

Kearnes, K., & Scher, G. (1988). The generalization of response elaboration training. In T. Prescott (Ed.), *Clinical aphasiology conference proceedings* (Vol. 18, pp. 223–245). Boston: College-Hill.

LPAA Project Group. (2001). Life participation approach to aphasia. In R. Chapey (Ed.), *Language intervention strategies in aphasia and related neurogenic communication disorder* (4th ed., pp. 235–245). Philadelphia: Lippincott Williams & Wilkins.

Anomic Aphasia

Characteristics

Word finding difficulties, also referred to as anomia or lexical retrieval difficulty, accompany most types of aphasia. However, when the individual has a disproportionately greater difficulty naming than other language difficulties, it is referred to as anomic aphasia. This deficit becomes most noticeable when the individual attempts confrontation naming, that is, naming an entity when a visual image is presented. These individuals often use circumlocutions and are frustrated by their inability to name things. However, the inability to retrieve and name words can be severe enough to completely halt the flow of speech and severely restrict discourse. Other salient features of anomic aphasia include fluent speech with the exception of intermittent hesitations. This halt in the flow of fluent speech is a direct result of the word-finding problem. For most people with anomic aphasia, morphology, syntax, and auditory comprehension are normal.

Anomia is generally caused by damage to the left inferior temporal cortex. If the damage occurs in the posterior portion of the inferior temporal cortex, pure anomia is more likely to be observed. Pure anomia results when access to phonological word forms is impaired. If the damage occurs in the more anterior portion of the temporal lobe, then semantic anomia is noted. This type of anomia is a result of a degradation of semantic knowledge. It also has been reported that the more anterior the lesion, the more severe the anomia. There is some suggestion that if the lesion extends into more ante-rior regions, the anomia will worsen. This is due to a disconnection between the areas critical for access of phonological words forms and areas of preserved semantic knowledge (Antonucci, Beeson, & Rap-csak, 2004).

Although patients with lesions in the left tem-poral pole can experience deficits in retrieving proper names for people, they maintain the ability to recognize them. Larger lesions may further affect the ability to name and often include difficulty nam-ing animals and tools (Tranel et al, 1997).

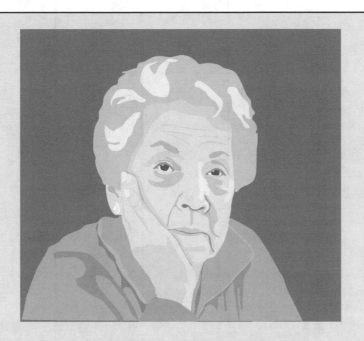

Case Scenario: Sophie

History and Physical (H & P): Sophie is a 63-year-old white female admitted to the ED via EMS; found on first floor of her home, sitting in a chair; lethargic, slurred speech; disoriented.

Past Medical History (PMH): Hypertension, hyperlipidemia, IDDM (insulin dependent diabetes mellitus), osteoarthritis.

Social History: Lives alone in two-story home, two blocks away from daughter and her family. Retired school teacher.

Surgical History: s/p right THR (total hip replacement); s/p angioplasty with stent in LAD (left anterior descending artery).

A Functional Analysis of Sophie's Aphasia

Sophie's ability to comprehend language in both verbal and written forms is within functional limits. Reading ability is normal at sentence and paragraph levels.

Language Expression	**Automatic Speech:** WFL for counting, days of the week, alphabet.	**Repetition Ability:** Normal repetition for words, phrases and sentences.	**Lexical Retrieval-Naming:** Impaired for confrontation naming and lexical retrieval during discourse; Circumlocutions noted.	**Conversational Ability:** WFL; however word finding difficulties impact speech fluency in conversation.	**Pragmatic Skills:** WFL	**Paraphasias:** None.
Speech	**Rate:** WFL	**Intelligibility:** WFL	**Prosody:** WFL	**Articulation:** WFL	**Fluency:** Impacted by word-finding difficulty.
Auditory Comprehension	**Answering Yes/No Questions:** WFL	**Executing Commands:** WFL	**Understanding Stories & Paragraphs:** WNL	**Understanding Conversational Speech:** Comprehension for sentences and discourse is WFL.	**Identifying Objects & their Functions:** WNL
Reading	**Word-level Comprehension:** WFL	**Sentence-level Comprehension:** WFL	**Oral Reading:** WFL	**Oral Spelling:** Letter substitutions noted in minimal pairs, e.g., mat for hat.
Written Expression	**Copying:** WFL	**Writing to Dictation:** WFL	**Self-generated:** Affected by word-finding difficulty.	**Written Spelling:** WFL for basic words.	**Drawing:** WFL
Cognition	**Attention/Concentration:** WFL	**Visuospatial Skills:** WFL	**Memory:** Long-term memory and working memory intact for procedural, semantic, and episodic systems.	**Executive Functions:** WFL
Behavioral Symptoms	**Alertness:** WFL	**Deficit awareness:** Keen awareness of deficits.	**Frustration:** Demonstrates extreme frustration with inability to retrieve desired words.	**Emotional Lability:** None.	**Current Personality Characteristics:** Pleasant and apologetic for her word-finding problems.

Figure 4–8. Diagnostic profile for Sophie.

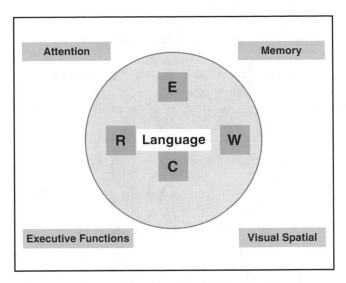

Figure 4–9. ALD Target Model for Sophie.

Her confrontational naming ability and word finding during discourse remain a challenge. However, Sophie can express herself to make her needs and wants known, even though she has a tendency to use circumlocutions to convey ideas. Speech rate and prosody are normal and intelligibility is good but fluency is impacted by her word-finding difficulties. Consequently, Sophie has many pauses and self-correcting attempts during telephone conversations an in public encounters, for example, shopping, banking, and managing public transportation exchanges.

Sophie's writing skills are good. She can write sentences but has some lexical retrieval difficulty in this domain as well. When she cannot think of a needed word she may ask the listener for help as she struggles. Although this can be an effective compensatory strategy, it is not always practical in public venues. Therefore, this causes more frustration for Sophie in that she knows she can find the means to express her ideas, but cannot readily use them in certain public scenarios.

Cognitively, Sophie displays good attention to tasks and can concentrate, especially if the task is of interest to her. Her memory skills for her ADL needs appear to be functioning within normal limits and she is able to recall basic information from events in the recent and distant past. She recalls how to cook her favorite meals and is able to manage her money and pay bills. Planning and judgment appear to be intact for common household tasks and chores, making appointments, and organizing her day. Sophie maintains a vibrant social network with her family and friends who are supportive of her rehabilitation goals. Although she is keenly aware of her deficits, she maintains a pleasant demeanor and continues to improve her functional communication skills by being actively engaged in her therapy program.

Critical Thinking/Learning Activity

- People with anomic aphasia can be classified into treatment categories that are semantically based, phonologically based, and self-cued (Boyle, 2004).
- How would you attempt to determine the most beneficial treatment for your patient?
- What will you use to support semantic and phonemic cuing?
- Which of Sophie's strengths can you use to promote word finding (lexical retrieval)?
- How will you advance Sophie's conversational skills with a variety of communication partners?
- Do you view Sophie's word finding difficulties as a receptive or expressive deficit? Explain.

Treatment Considerations

Some general therapeutic objectives and techniques applicable to Sophie's deficit profile include:

- Improve lexical retrieval to request information and assistance using semantic feature analysis (SFA). For each word she cannot access, the category to which the item belongs, its action, physical properties, location, and associated features, will be sought.
- Increase engagement in conversation with designated people using comprehension tasks that facilitate oral naming. For word finding difficulties, supportive pictures, and a written list of functional words to view will be provided.
- Make needs and wants known with semantic and phonemic self-cueing to increase word finding. Provide words following circumlocutions.
- Based on Sophie's needed activities of daily living (ADL), make her needs and wants known for use during conversation and begin facilitating their use in functional contexts.

Some Therapeutic Options

- Response-Contingent Small Step Treatment (RCSST) (Bollinger & Stout, 1976).
- Promoting Aphasic Communicative Effectiveness (PACE) (Li et al., 1988).
- Semantic Feature Analysis (SFA) (Coelho, McHugh, & Boyle, 2000).
- Semantic Cueing Treatment (SCT) (Wambaugh et al., 2001).
- Phonological Cueing Treatment (PCT) (Wambaugh et al., 2001).
- Cognitive Neuropsychological Models of Lexical Processing (Raymer & Rothi, 2001).
- Semantic Judgment Questions, Written Word to Picture Matching, and Naming to Definitions (Drew et al., 1999).

References

Antonucci, S. M., Beeson, P. M., & Rapcsak, S. Z. (2004). Anomia in patients with left inferior temporal lobe lesions. *Aphasiology, 18*, 543–554.

Bollinger, R. L., & Stout, C. E. (1976). Response-contingent small-step treatment: Performance-based communication intervention. *Journal of Speech and Hearing Disorders, 41*, 40–51.

Boyle, M. (2004). Semantic feature analysis: The evidence for treating lexical impairments in aphasia. *Aphasia: Treatment for lexical and sentence production skills.* Rockville, MD: American Speech-Language-Hearing Association.

Coelho, C. S., McHugh, R., & Boyle, M. (2000). Semantic feature analysis as a treatment for aphasic dysnomia: A replication. *Aphasiology, 14*, 133–142.

Drew, R. L., & Thompson, C. K. (1999). Model-based semantic treatment for naming deficits in aphasia. *Journal of Speech, Language, and Hearing Research, 4*, 972–990.

Li, E. C., Kitselman, K., Dusatko, D., & Spinelli, C. (1988). The efficacy of PACE in the remediation of naming deficits. *Journal of Communication Disorders, 21*, 491–503.

Raymer, A. M., & Rothi, L. J. G. (2001). Cognitive approaches to impairments of word comprehension and production. In R. Chapey (Ed.), *Language intervention strategies in aphasia and related neurogenic communication disorders* (4th ed., pp. 524–550). Baltimore: Lippincott, Williams & Wilkins.

Tranel, D., Logan, C. G., Frank, R. J., & Damasio, A. R. (1997). Explaining category-related effects in the retrieval of conceptual and lexical knowledge for concrete entities: Operationalization and analysis of factors. *Neuropsychologia, 35*, 1329–1339.

Wambaugh, J. L., Linebaugh, C. W., Doyle, P. J., Martinez, A. L., Kalinyak-Flisar, M., & Spencer, K. A. (2001). Effects of two cueing treatments on lexical retrieval treatments in aphasic speakers with different levels of deficit. *Aphasiology, 15*, 933–950.

Chapter 5

OTHER APHASIC SYNDROMES

Subcortical Aphasia

Characteristics

The advances in neuroradiologic imaging and in the understanding of the role of subcortical structures in language support a more serious consideration of the subcortical aphasias (Kent, 2004). Understanding subcortical aphasias can be challenging even for the most seasoned clinicians. Part of this difficulty lies in the terminology of the brain structures involved. Therefore, it makes the most sense to start there.

According to Webb, Adler, and Love (2008), subcortical aphasia became a new category of aphasia as better imaging techniques became available. Studying thalamic hemorrhage without cerebral cortex involvement and ischemic infarction of the thalamus via advanced imaging studies were instrumental in establishing the disorder. The subcortical aphasias are often divided into thalamic and nonthalamic types (Davis, 2007; Nadeau & Rothi, 2001). Subcortical aphasias are observed when there is vascular damage resulting in neuronal death which occurs in the left hemisphere below the cortex. The primary subcortical areas include:

- The internal capsule (white matter pathways)
- The basal ganglia
- The thalamus

The internal capsule is a passageway for motor and sensory fiber tracts and is located between the thalamus and the lenticular nuclei. The caudate nucleus and the putamen make up the lenticular nuclei, and together the caudate and the putamen are called the striatum. The lenticular nuclei comprise a part of the basal ganglia. The capsulostriatum comprises the internal capsule, the caudate nucleus, and the putamen. It is in the region of the capsulostriatum that most subcortical infracts generally occur.

The role of the nonthalamic structures in normal and impaired language processes is controversial. The actual controversy lies not in the fact that it is possible to sustain language impairment due to lesions in this region; it is the variability in nature and degree of those impairments that raises some questions (Kennedy & Murdoch, 1993; Nadeau & Crosson, 1997). Some authors have reported differences in the language impairment of those patients with anterior striatocapsular lesions versus those with posterior striatocapsular lesions (Cappa, Cavallotti, Guidotti, Papagno, & Vignolo, 1983; Murdoch, Thompson, Fraser, & Harrison, 1986; Naeser, Helm-Estabrooks, Levine, Laughlin, & Geschwind, 1982). However, Kennedy and Murdoch (1993) described cases in which the differences in language difficulties could not be attributed to an anterior-posterior distinction, leaving this controversy unresolved.

The basal ganglia and thalamus are connected to the cerebral cortex by a series of white matter circuits called the *cortico-striato-pallido-thalamo-cortical loops*. The thalamus is a nucleus located deep in the cerebrum. It is connected to motor, sensory, and association areas of the cortex. It is a primary relay station for information entering and leaving the cerebral cortex. For example, a hallmark of thalamic aphasia is poor attention. This is thought to be due to a lesion in the white fibers connecting the thalamus to the prefrontal cortex (Davis, 2007, p. 48). Aphasias due to thalamic lesions are better understood and better documented compared with aphasias that are due to nonthalamic subcortical lesions. A reason for this discrepancy is that the nonthalamic lesions had not been visible on imaging studies (Chapey, 2001, p. 460). The clinical profile for thalamic aphasia is more unitary and, consequently, a clinician would be able to determine the existence of a thalamic aphasia more easily. For a thorough and succinct review of the subcortical aphasias see Kent (2004) (Table 5–1).

These two types of subcortical aphasia have critical differences with the exception of spared repetition which is preserved in both. To differentiate characteristics of subcortical aphasias, individuals that have striatocapsular involvement and white matter paraventricular lesions generally experience a lack of speech fluency, literal (phonemic) paraphasias, but generally preserved comprehension and naming. Individuals with thalamic aphasia generally experience fluent speech output but have impaired comprehension, naming and verbal (semantic) paraphasias (Kuljic-Obradovic, 2003) (Figure 5–1).

Table 5–1. Characteristics of Thalamic and Nonthalamic Subcortical Aphasias

Thalamic Aphasia	Nonthalamic Aphasia
Fluent speech	Impaired speech fluency
Impaired confrontation naming	Confrontation naming is good
Repetition is preserved	Repetition is preserved
Impaired auditory comprehension	Auditory comprehension is preserved
Normal speech articulation	Phonological disorder
Normal grammar	Grammar impairment
Semantic paraphasias and neologisms	Literal paraphasia

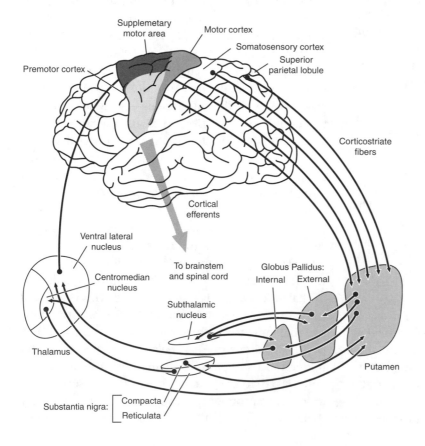

Figure 5–1. Subcortical pathways (Adapted from Bhatnagar, 2002, p. 256).

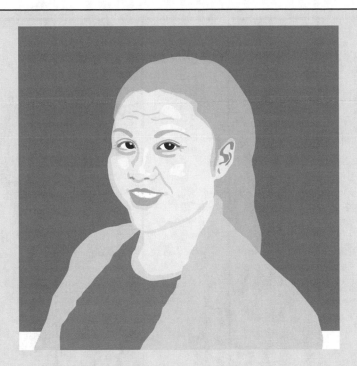

Case Scenario: Winnie

History and Physical (H & P): 63-year-old, right-handed, Vietnamese female, admitted to local hospital. Numbness in the right arm and shoulder; lethargy. On examination, her level of alertness was significantly reduced. Family brought her to the hospital describing her as "babbling and sleepy." Blood pressure in the ED was 130/85 and heart rate was 92. She did not seem to understand the questions asked of her.

Past Medical History (PMH): Winnie has no prior history of stroke. Her PMH includes hyperlipidemia and HTN. She is compliant with all medications.

Social History: Lives with her husband and her son and his family in a two-story row home in Philadelphia. Winnie speaks proficient English as a second language. She has been in the United States since 1977. Completed required schooling in South Vietnam.

Surgical History: Unremarkable.

A Functional Analysis of Winnie's Subcortical Aphasia

In the acute phase of the stroke, Winnie presented with extreme lethargy, often dozing off during the middle of a communicative interaction. Her lethargy complicates her already compromised ability to process auditory information, especially at the conversational level. It is important for the clinician to understand the impact that Winnie's level of alertness has on her auditory processing skills

Language Expression	**Automatic Speech:** WFL for counting, days of the week, alphabet with a verbal prompt to facilitate initiation.	**Repetition Ability:** WFL for words and sentences, however some paraphasias noted.	**Lexical Retrieval-Naming:** Confrontation naming is moderate-severely impaired.	**Conversational Ability:** Syntax WFL at sentence level. However, her lethargy and paraphasias complicate her functional discourse.	**Pragmatic Skills:** Affected by lethargy and difficulty maintaining the communication dyad. / **Paraphasias:** Semantic paraphasias present.
Speech	**Rate:** Slowed rate, hesitant speech.	**Intelligibility:** WFL	**Prosody:** Reduced intonation contours; may be secondary to lethargy.	**Articulation:** WFL	**Fluency:** Speech output is borderline fluent (6-8 words per utterance), with semantic paraphasias present.
Auditory Comprehension	**Answering Yes/No Questions:** Response accuracy affected by level of alertness.	**Executing Commands:** Able to execute one-step commands when alert.	**Understanding Stories & Paragraphs:** Impaired due to inability to maintain attention and concentration.	**Understanding Conversational Speech:** Severely impaired at the conversational level due to lethargy and inattentiveness	**Identifying Objects & their Functions:** Able to name and identify common objects when alert and attentive.
Reading	**Word-level Comprehension:** WFL for common words in large print.	**Sentence-level Comprehension:** Moderately impaired at the paragraph level due to lack of attention at the time of assessment.	**Oral Reading:** Reading aloud is slow and labored.	**Oral Spelling:** Some difficulty spelling commonly used words; may be secondary to problems with declarative memory.	
Written Expression	**Copying:** WFL	**Writing to Dictation:** Paragraphic errors noted.	**Self-generated:** Functional for ADL needs: signature, address, names of family.	**Written Spelling:** Paragraphic errors.	**Drawing:** Able to execute simple line drawings when alert.
Cognition	**Attention/Concentration:** Poor.	**Visuospatial Skills:** Functional but optimized with large print and pictures.	**Memory:** Declarative functioning is impaired; procedural motor memory for ADLs is impaired.	**Executive Functions:** Ability to solve problems associated with ADLs varies based on the complexity of those tasks due to her concentration and memory	
Behavioral Symptoms	**Alertness:** Lethargic, but not oppositional. Cooperative, as able.	**Deficit awareness:** She is aware of her communication deficits as indicated by yes/no responses to questions.	**Frustration:** None noted at the time of assessment.	**Emotional Lability:** None noted.	**Current Personality Characteristics:** Cannot determine at the time of assessment due to lethargy.

Figure 5–2. Diagnostic profile for Winnie.

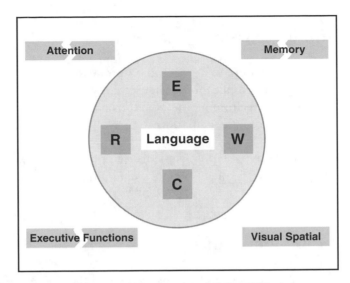

Figure 5–3. ALD Target Model for Winnie.

and to adjust the therapy accordingly. Although Winnie speaks fluently, her speech is characterized by numerous semantic paraphasias. From a functional perspective, Winnie's paraphasic output can be circumvented if the listener uses the context of the exchange to facilitate appropriate word selection. She is very aware of her receptive and expressive deficits, but appears almost indifferent to them. Reading is impaired at the paragraph level, but is functional at the word and phrase levels. The clinician may want to consider using Winnie's reading skills at the word/phrase level to promote growth in other deficit areas. Since the written word is static, and not fleeting like the speech signal, Winnie processes and attends better to this type of stimuli. This can help her process information for communication purposes. Therapeutically, the clinician can pair the written word with the speech signal to optimize Winnie's comprehension of more difficult material, if necessary. Winnie's difficulty maintaining attention affects all areas of cognition. To complicate matters, Winnie demonstrates memory deficits for declarative functioning. In other words, her procedural motor memory for activities such as dressing, cooking, and grooming are less impaired than her ability to talk about them. This is an instance where the written word and/or pictures can facilitate procedural functioning. Visuospatial skills are functional but are optimized with large print and pictures. Using simple drawings and bold print as well as pictures with emotional valence are suggested. Winnie's ability to solve problems associated with her ADLs will vary based on her procedural memory and the number of steps involved completing the task. Therefore, Winnie may not be able to manage some of her ADLs such as cooking independently. However, every patient is different so this admonishment is merely cautionary. Her functional profile will change in a positive direction as her level of alertness increases.

Critical Thinking/Learning Activity

1. What would you do to determine if Winnie's processing deficit is an aphasic symptom or simply a complication of her lethargy?
2. Why will Winnie benefit from multimodality cueing?
3. Which of Winnie's strengths can you use to facilitate improvement in her weaker areas?
4. Given her symptoms, what type of subcortical aphasia does Winnie exhibit?
5. Why would you want to facilitate Winnie's self-monitoring of her speech output?

Treatment Considerations

Winnie's lethargy will affect her ability to participate in the therapy, especially in the acute phase. Therefore, the clinician's first task is to arouse the patient to a level of alertness (LOA) that supports her ability to participate in therapy. Daily monitoring of her LOA is essential for determining when to initiate direct intervention. Noting the changes in her gaze, eye contact, facial expression, and so forth, are practical ways to monitor her LOA prior to each session. The three primary areas that need to be addressed in this case in order to optimize Winnie's functional communication are:

- Word retrieval
- Auditory comprehension
- Semantic paraphasias

Once her LOA supports direct treatment, consider the following:

- It is important to demonstrate patience. Winnie may need more time to process a simple command and respond.
- Supplement auditorily presented information with pictures and words in large print format. This will optimize her response by engaging her visual attention system.
- Train Winnie in the use of self-cuing strategies to compensate for her word retrieval deficit. For example, you can teach her how to use phonemic self-cues to facilitate word retrieval. You can also instruct her in self-cuing with descriptive cues, that is, describe the object's characteristics, but this may be more difficult for her due to her semantic paraphasias.
- Contextual cues methods can be effective, that is, avoid confrontation naming approaches but use and talk about objects in a functional context related to a purpose. For example, talk about getting dressed for the day and facilitate discussion about the necessary items needed to accomplish this activity of daily living. Consider co-treating with occupational therapy during morning ADL treatment.

■ To develop the ability to self-monitor speech output is essential in a patient presenting with semantic paraphasias. This can be very challenging for the clinician depending on the severity of the auditory comprehension impairment. However, there are a few things that you can do to optimize this function. First, always use an auditory alerting signal to increase Winnie's attention to the incoming signal. This can be a tap on the desk or even a statement such as "Winnie, listen." If you ask Winnie an open-ended question such as, "What do you put on your feet?" and she answers "hat" instead of "shoe" try the following method. First, ask her if "hat" was correct. If she says, "No," you can facilitate the target word with a phonemic cue. On the other hand, if she said, "Yes," indicating her inability to self-monitor, then provides the correct word accompanied by a picture or real object of the target. The clinician can heighten her awareness of her errors by feeding back the incorrect word choices with a questioning intonation. Be sure to instruct Winnie to "listen to herself very carefully" so that she can pick out her incorrect word choices. She would then use her self-cuing techniques for naming that you trained. Notice how self-monitoring and naming are entwined in this case and in many others that you will encounter.

Some Therapeutic Options

■ Schuell's Stimulation Approach to Rehabilitation (Duffy & Coelho, 2001).
■ Cognitive Stimulation: Stimulation of recognition/comprehension, memory and thinking (Chapey, 2001).
■ Any program that works on parallel distributed processing (PDP) model of language function (Chapey, 2001).

References

Bhatnagar, S. C. (2002). *Neuroscience for the study of communicative disorders* (2nd ed.). Baltimore: Lippincott Williams & Wilkins.

Cappa, S. F., Cavallotti, G., Guidotti, M., Papagno, C., & Vignolo, L. A. (1983). Subcortical aphasia: Two clinical-CT scan correlation studies. *Cortex, 19,* 227–241.

Chapey, R. (Ed.). (2001). *Language intervention strategies in aphasia and related neurogenic communication disorders* (4th ed.). Philadelphia: Lippincott Williams & Wilkins.

Davis, G. A. (2007). Cognitive pragmatics of language disorders in adults. *Seminars in Speech and Language, 28*(2), 111–121.

Duffy, J. R., & Coelho, C. A. (2001). Schuell's stimulation approach to rehabilitation. In R. Chapey (Ed.), *Language intervention strategies in aphasia and related neurogenic communication disorders* (4th ed., pp. 403–449). Philadelphia: Lippincott Williams & Wilkins.

Kennedy, M., & Murdoch, B. (1993). Chronic aphasia subsequent to striato-capsular and thalamic lesions in the left hemisphere. *Brain and Language, 44*(3), 284–295.

Kent, R. D. (Ed.). (2004). *The MIT encyclopedia of communication disorders.* Cambridge, MA: Massachusetts Institute of Technology.

Kuljic-Obradovic, D. C. (2003). Subcortical aphasia: Three different language disorder syndromes? *European Journal of Neurology, 10*(4), 445–448.

Nadeau, S., & Crosson, B. (1997). Subcortical aphasia, *Brain and Language, 58*(3), 355–402.

Nadeau, S. E., & Rothi, L. J. G. (2001). Rehabilitation of subcortical aphasia. In R. Chapey (Ed.), *Language intervention strategies in aphasia and related neurogenic communication disorders* (4th ed.). Philadelphia: Lippincott Williams & Wilkins.

Naeser, M., Alexander, M., Helm-Estabrooks, N., Levine, N., Laughlin S., & Geschwind, N. (1982). Aphasia with predominantly subcortical lesion sites: Description of three capsular/putaminal aphasia syndromes. *Neurology, 39*(1), 2–14.

Webb, W. G., Adler, R. K., & Love, R. J. (2008). *Neurology for the speech-language pathologist.* St. Louis, MO: Mosby Elsevier.

Primary Progressive Aphasia

Characteristics

Primary progressive aphasia (PPA) is of unknown etiology and is progressive and currently untreatable. It is a form of dementia characterized by a degeneration of the language functions, reading, writing, speaking, and comprehension. Onset is insidious with a gradual and slow decline. PPA can be associated with other neurologic symptoms and these include: dysarthria, dysphagia, oral apraxia, right central facial droop or weakness, right extremity weakness, and limb apraxia (Kavrie & Duffy, 1994; McNeil, 1998). On autopsy, other pathologic diagnoses have been associated with PPA. These include progressive supranuclear palsy, corticobasal degeneration, corticonigral degeneration, amyotrophic lateral sclerosis (ALS), and Creutzfeldt-Jacob disease. (Mandel, Alexander, & Carpenter, 1989). It is also known as a slowly progressive aphasia. Initially, memory and other cognitive abilities, as well as personality, remain intact. However, over time, other mental faculties begin to deteriorate. This is considered a precursor to dementia or Alzheimer's disease, and onset tends to be in younger people with symptoms often beginning in the fifth decade of life. The average age of onset tends to be around 60 years. Incidence is higher in males than females. The site of degeneration in PPA is usually in the left fronto-temporal-parietal region (perisylvian). Patients with early signs of PPA initially present with word finding difficulties in both speaking and writing tasks. They also demonstrate semantic word substitutions (*car/bus*); phonemic word substitutions (*pin/bin*); and circumlocutions (*I went to the place that you buy the paper*, referring to "I went to the newsstand"). In the early stages of this process, they can maintain normal activities of daily living because memory and other cognitive skills are still intact. These patients have difficulty following conversations and participating in groups. They have diminished use of expressive language and their verbal output can be void of meaning. Later in the disease process they demonstrate difficulty with numbers and performing simple mathematical calculations. PPA is often known as a cortical degeneration syndrome (Caselli, 1995). Research has found that that any type of aphasic symptoms is possible and that individuals at earlier stages tend to sound fluent. However, as the disease progress individuals tend to sound more nonfluent (Weintraub, Rubin, & Mesulam, 1990).

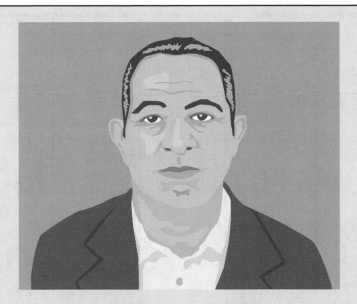

Case Scenario: Luis

History and Physical (H & P): 58-year-old, right-handed, Hispanic male, taken to physician's office by daughter who complained of his speech and language difficulties; right extremity clumsiness; no gross physical weakness; noted difficulty with word finding; articulation of speech unclear with sound substitutions. Luis is cognitively intact according to his daughter.

Past Medical History (PMH): Patient complain of language difficulty over 2-years; previous imaging studies have identified focal atrophy in language zone; slight HTN (hypertension) but otherwise in good health.

Social History: Widower with 1 adult daughter; lives with daughter in 2-bedroom apartment; worked as a retail clerk at a local home improvement store (duties now limited to stock clerk due to difficulty communicating). Patient is cognitively intact and does not believe he is having any difficulty with his mental abilities; independent in most ADLs (activities of daily living) at home and at work.

Surgical History: Hernia repair 10 years prior.

A Functional Analysis of Luis' Primary Progressive Aphasia

Luis' ability to understand language is intact. He enjoys interacting with others in conversation although he is often frustrated by his word finding difficulties and reduced speech intelligibility. Despite his frustration and looming depression, Luis remains motivated to improve his functional communication. He is aware of his speech and language difficulties and tries to self-correct; however, his family is skeptical about his true understanding of the progressive nature of this disease process. Cognitively, Luis demonstrates good attentional skills and is

Language Expression

- **Automatic Speech:** WFL for counting, reciting the alphabet, stating days and months of the year.
- **Repetition Ability:** Repetition of multisyllabic words is impaired.
- **Lexical Retrieval-Naming:** Difficulty with lexical retrieval. Often states he knows what he wants to say but can't find the words.
- **Conversational Ability:** Unable to carry on a fluent conversation.
- **Pragmatic Skills:** Understands the rules of conversation but his word-finding, and verbal non-fluency affect his pragmatic language.
- **Paraphasias:** Semantic paraphasias are present with similarly categorized words often substituted.

Speech

- **Rate:** Slow rate of speech.
- **Intelligibility:** WFL in known and unknown contexts.
- **Prosody:** Aprosodic speech with inappropriate inflection, rhythm, and stress.
- **Articulation:** Mild spastic dysarthria characterized by articulatory distortions and dysprosody.
- **Fluency:** Diminished use of expressive language. Average phrase length varies but is generally 4 words or less.

Auditory Comprehension

- **Answering Yes/No Questions:** WFL for concrete and personal questions.
- **Executing Commands:** WFL
- **Understanding Stories & Paragraphs:** Comprehension for words and sentences is relatively intact. Paragraph length material is good for concrete concepts.
- **Understanding Conversational Speech:** Relatively intact; however comprehension is impaired at the conversational level with multiple conversational partners.
- **Identifying Objects & their Functions:** WFL

Reading

- **Word-level Comprehension:** WFL
- **Sentence-level Comprehension:** WFL
- **Oral Reading:** Oral reading is WFL but deteriorates as word length increases.
- **Oral Spelling:** Able to spell common words when given the word verbally.

Written Expression

- **Copying:** WFL for common words.
- **Writing to Dictation:** WFL for basic words.
- **Self-generated:** Characterized by semantic and phonological paraphasias.
- **Written Spelling:** Paragraphic.
- **Drawing:** WFL

Cognition

- **Attention/Concentration:** WFL
- **Visuospatial Skills:** Can read print and identify photos and pictures.
- **Memory:** Procedural, semantic and episodic WFL for ADLs.
- **Executive Functions:** Problem solving skills and reasoning intact for ADL needs.

Behavioral Symptoms

- **Alertness:** WFL
- **Deficit awareness:** Aware of speech production and language difficulties and attempts to self-correct.
- **Frustration:** Very frustrated and becoming depressed. Motivated to improve.
- **Emotional Lability:** None noted.
- **Current Personality Characteristics:** Pleasant, sociable, and motivated to improve.

Figure 5–4. Diagnostic profile for Luis.

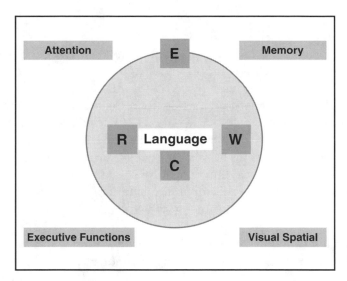

Figure 5–5. ALD Target Model for Luis.

very willing to work in therapy. His episodic, semantic, and procedural memory systems for ADLs are functioning within normal limits at this time, based on his activities in the home. Visuospatial skills appear intact and he is able to read print and identify photos and pictures. Currently, Luis demonstrates normal problem-solving skills and can reason to make appropriate decisions during the day at home. For example, Luis can dress and groom himself and can prepare a simple meal independently. He still plays poker and rummy with his close friends regularly, with an adaptive tray for card organization and manipulation.

Critical Thinking/Learning Activity

■ Given that this patient has articulation difficulties and oral apraxia, what information in his history helps to differentiate apraxia from dysarthria?
■ In what ways does this patient resemble a nonfluent aphasic?
■ What would be your rationale for providing treatment or not providing treatment to Luis? Select a position and defend it based on the information about PPA and Luis' profile.
■ What kind of counseling and education would you provide to Luis' family? Please include content information as well as emotional support.

Treatment Considerations

Luis is strong in many communication areas. His auditory comprehension and reading comprehension are near normal. He is able to understand linguistic material at the paragraph level and is able to follow a conversation with one communication partner. Luis is able to count, name the days of the week and the months of the year, which are important for ADL needs. His sentence length is four words or fewer. Luis' primary weaknesses are his dysarthria and his word-finding difficulties. These two deficits combine to reduce Luis' ability to be a functional communicator in all social contexts. However, a complication in Luis' case that is not found in the other aphasic syndromes is that PPA is progressive and degenerative. Because Luis has a strong social support network, is motivated to engage in treatment, and has other cognitive strengths (attention and memory), treatment should be considered. Due to the nature of Luis' profile, the clinician needs to have multiple foci of treatment, which are:

- Maintaining functional communication over the long term of the disease process, as possible, using any modality available to Luis.
- Building on Luis' stronger language skills to optimize his functional communication in the short term.
- Establishing an alternative communication method, for example, gesture or augmentative devices.
- Train Luis in the use of compensatory speech strategies to increase his speech intelligibility in known and unknown contexts.
- Facilitate word finding ability to reduce frustration and increase verbal fluency
- Provide ongoing family counseling and education regarding the goals and procedures of therapy across the course of the disease.

Some Therapeutic Options

- Lexical-Semantic Activation Inhibition Treatment (L-SAIT) (McNeil, Small, Masterson, & Fossett, 1995).
- Semantic Feature Analysis (SFA) (Boyle & Coelho, 1995).
- AAC devices and software.
- Life Participation Approach to Aphasia (LPAA) (Chapey, Duchan, Elman, Garcia, Kagan, Lyon, & Simmons-Mackie, 2008).
- Speech conservation strategies to optimize intelligibility.
- Back to the Drawing Board (Morgan & Helm-Estabrooks, 1987).
- Support group for patients and families dealing with PPA

References

Boyle, M., & Coelho, C. A. (1995). Application of semantic feature analysis as a treatment for aphasic dysnomia. *American Journal of Speech-Language Pathology, 4,* 94–98.

Caselli, R. J. (1995). Focal and asymmetric cortical degeneration syndromes. *Neurologist, 1*(1), 1–19.

Chapey, R., Duchan, J. F., Elman, R. J., Garcia, L. J., Kagan, A., Lyon, J. G., et al. (2008). Life-participation approach to aphasia: A statement of values for the future. In R. Chapey (Ed.), *Language intervention strategies in aphasia and related neurogenic communication disorders* (5th ed.). Philadelphia: Wolters Kluwer/Lippincott Williams & Wilkins.

Kavrie, S. H., & Duffy, J. R. (1994). *Primary progressive apraxia of speech*. Paper presented at the annual convention of the American Speech-Language-Hearing Association, New Orleans, LA.

Mandel, A., Alexander, M., & Carpenter, S. (1989). Creutzfeldt-Jakob disease presenting as isolated aphasia. *Neurology, 39*, 55.

McNeil, M. R. (1998). The case of the lawyer's lugubrious language: Dysarthria plus primary progressive aphasia or dysarthria plus dementia? *Seminars in Speech and Language, 19*(1), 49–57.

McNeil, M. R., & Duffy, J. R. (2001). Primary progressive aphasia. In R. Chapey (Ed.), *Language intervention strategies in aphasia and related neurogenic communication disorders* (4th ed.). Philadelphia: Lippincott Williams & Wilkins.

McNeil, M. R., Small, S. L., Masterson, R. J., & Fossett, T. R. D. (1995). Behavioral and pharmacological treatment of lexical-semantic deficits in a single patient with primary progressive aphasia. *American Journal of Speech-Language Pathology, 4*, 76–87.

Morgan, A. L., & Helm-Estabrooks, N. (1987). Back to the drawing board: A treatment program for nonverbal aphasic patients. *Clinical Aphasiology, 16*, 34–39.

Weintraub, S., Rubin, N. P., & Mesulam, M. M. (1990). Primary progressive aphasia: Longitudinal course, neurological profile and language features. *Archives of Neurology, 47*(12), 1329–1335.

Acquired Alexia and Agraphia

Characteristics

In order to explain the processes of alexia it is necessary to provide the reader with some fundamental knowledge of normal reading. The goal in reading is for words to be comprehended via print, yet it is possible for a person to read without obtaining any meaning from the text. However, initially, in order to read with meaning, one must connect letters to sounds that blend together to form words or read a word as a whole unit. Words then activate semantic knowledge and the written text can be understood. Once this process becomes automatic, an individual typically reads fluently via whole word

recognition. The following sections introduce the three routes of normal reading. With this knowledge the reader should better comprehend the processes of phonological alexia, surface alexia and deep alexia.

Characteristics of Normal Reading

The visual information presented as words on the page is projected to the extrastriate cortex in the right occipital lobe. Early visual analysis (EVA) of words can be interpreted via three types of reading routes: *phonic, direct,* and *lexical.* For the phonic route, there is an EVA for letters. This requires learning abstract symbols as graphemes (written letters corresponding to sounds in a language). Here, visual information travels via the corpus callosum to the left temporal lobe for phonemic coding. After the letters are parsed or separated for individual coding, graphemes are connected with phonemes (sounds for the letters) to be blended into words. Auditory cues help decipher the word through the angular gyrus and the supramarginal gyrus. For example, children learning to read the word CAT via the *phonic route* will learn the corresponding sound for each letter. After the letters are parsed for individual coding, they are blended together to sound out the word CAT and connect it with its real-life object. If the *direct route* is used, the EVA works with whole words. Whole word recognition travels to Broca's area through the arcuate fasciculus. The word can then be read aloud. If the *lexical route* is used, the EVA works with a *morphological decomposer.* In this context, for example, a young child learning to read the word *teacher* will decompose the *–er* morpheme as the lexical marker for "one who teaches." Another example of morphological decomposition is in the morph *–ology,* meaning "the study of," being separated from the morph attached to it— rheumatology, biology, morphology, and so forth. Therefore in the lexical route, these words produce semantic representations for comprehension of the written word. Ultimately, the insular cortex automatizes the process to permit rapid automatic word recognition with comprehension. Information is sent to the frontal lobes for output, that is, reading aloud (Duffy & Geschwind, 1985). It is important to understand that the phonic, direct, and lexical routes are operating simultaneously in a normal, fluent reader.

Alexia

An individual can have a breakdown in any of the three reading routes. A breakdown in the phonic route produces a phonological alexia; a breakdown in the direct route may lead to surface alexia; and a breakdown in the lexical route may lead to a deep alexia. *Graphemes*, or letters corresponding to the sounds of a language, are converted to sounds which can be read. The graphemes also activate the semantic system when read and understood. A foundational process necessary for reading and writing requires the ability to turn sounds into letters, that is, phonemes into graphemes, so that the meaning of a word can be activated, and thus understood by the reader.

According to Chapey (2001), the semantic system is at the central point in the reading and writing process (p. 573). She depicts both *lexical-semantic* and *sublexical* routes for both reading and writing. There are three primary routes that can activate the semantic system: the *visual representation* (object or picture), the *phonological input lexicon route* (sound-to-letter correspondence), and the *graphemic input lexicon route* (letter-to-sound correspondence). The visual representation route uses a visual object or picture to convey meaning. This direct path allows a person to see an image, for example, a flower, and know what it is. The phonological input lexicon route converts a phoneme into a letter which can be written and read. This does not guarantee meaning. The third route is the graphemic input lexicon. Letters in print correspond to sounds which can then be read. This activates the semantic system when the word is understood.

Neurologic disease or damage can impair processing of the reading-writing system so that comprehension and production of written words are no longer possible. Word length, word frequency, and the concrete nature of the word itself all contribute to the problems individuals have with reading.

There are two broad classifications of alexia: central and peripheral. Central alexia is found in the presence of aphasia. Normal readers read by sound and by sight, that is, by sounding out words and by recognizing words. For example, recognizing the word *the*, yet sounding out the word *bibliography*, based on sound pattern and spelling rules in English.

For a person with central alexia, there is impairment in using these two reading routes, producing the observable alexia. Table 5–2 provides a review of the types of *central alexia*, damage incurred, and salient features (Beeson & Hillis, 2001). Table 5–3 provides an overview of *peripheral alexia profiles*.

Peripheral alexia is defined as reading difficulties that occur without a concomitant aphasia. There are five types of peripheral alexia. A patient with global alexia reads very slowly and/or inaccurately, but can recognize letters, and numbers can be spared. A patient with pure alexia cannot read words and needs a letter-by-letter strategy to do so. When the patient spells the word aloud, reading comprehension is better. Hemianopic alexia is characterized by an inability to read prefixes and suffixes; and in a neglect alexia, prefixes are more in error than suffixes. The patient presenting with an attentional alexia will crowd letters together and merge words.

Leff, Crewes, Plant, Scott, Kennard, and Wise (2001) investigated single-word reading in patients with hemianopsia and pure alexia. Pure alexia has been defined as a severe disturbance in reading comprehension with linguistically accurate writing, normal oral spelling, and the absence of aphasia or dementia. Pure alexia results from an inability to map letters in a familiar sequence to mental representation of the word. For those with pure alexia, it is a right hemianopsia that may impede single-word reading due to an inability to see letters at the end of a word. The work of Leff et al. (2001) demonstrated patients with hemianopic alexia activated the left occipitotemporal junction although there was lack of input from the ipsilateral primary and prestriate visual cortex. Therefore, it was determined that destruction of the left occipitotemporal junction can result in a severe impairment of word recognition or pure alexia. It has been noted that alexia resulting from a middle cerebral artery stroke accompanies a generalized language disorder. A person with a mild naming deficit may also have pure alexia if it is associated with a left posterior cerebral artery infarct. Although rare, there have been reported cases of pure alexia without hemianopsia and for those individuals there was often a generalized language disorder (Iragui & Kritchevsky, 1991; Sinn & Blanken, 1999).

Table 5–2. Types of Central Alexia

Central Alexia	Damage	Salient Features
Phonological Alexia (reads by sight)	▪ Cannot sound out the phonemes associated with the graphemes so the meaning of words cannot be obtained (impaired graphemic input lexicon)	▪ Cannot sound out words ▪ Sound-symbol disassociation ▪ Relies on word shape to facilitate reading ▪ Uses memory as a strategy to facilitate reading. ▪ May benefit from retraining letter-to-sound correspondence
Surface Alexia (reads by sound)	▪ Impaired representation of translating the way the word looks to its meaning (graphemic input lexicon) ▪ A variant of this is difficulty noted when the person regularizes irregularly spelled words (impaired phonological output lexicon)	▪ Visually perceived words that were once familiar are no longer identifiable or meaningful ▪ Relies heavily on sounding out words letter by letter to facilitate reading ▪ Irregular words such as "rhythm" are difficult ▪ Has difficulty making reading "automatic" ▪ May regularize a word that is spelled irregularly ("yacht" may be read as "yet") ▪ Typically seen in individuals with progressive language deterioration or other neurodegenerative processes ▪ May benefit from work on phoneme-grapheme pairs to sound out letters in words (establish a key word for each letter) ▪ High-frequency words are easier ▪ Written words may cue speech output (reading aloud)
Deep Alexia (both sound and sight routes damaged)	▪ Difficulty recognizing written words, understanding their meaning, and sounding out words using letter-to-sound conversions (semantics and letter-to-sound correspondence impairment)	▪ There may be semantic errors in oral reading, visual errors for words that look similar, and substitutions of words within a word class ▪ Nouns are more easily read compared with adjectives due to their conceptual saliency ▪ Adjectives are easier than verbs and verbs are easier than function words ▪ Abstract, low-frequency words are most difficult ▪ Error words may be linked to the target word through association (e.g., reading *dinner* as food). ▪ May benefit from methods to associate sounds with letters

Agraphia

Agraphia (or dysgraphia) is a term used to indicate a writing impairment. Agraphia reflects a lexical-semantic breakdown. Links between written words and their meanings are impaired. Letters and sound associations are often affected. Deep agraphia involves impairment with written semantics. High-frequency words, high-imagery words, and nouns are often written with greater ease. Those with deep agraphia

Table 5–3. Types of Peripheral Alexia

Peripheral Subtype	Damage	Salient Features
Global	- Left ventrolateral occipitotemporal cortex (VLOT) or splenium of corpus callosum	- Slow or inaccurate letter naming - Can recognize letters and often numbers
Pure Alexia (Alexia without Agraphia)	- Left VLOT or connections - Can see the letters but cannot identify the group of letters as a visual word with meaning (impaired access to graphemic input lexicon)	- Slow and inaccurate reading, short words are easier - Cannot recognize strings of letters as words although knows the letters - Writing is intact - Spelling the word helps identify it - Usually benefits from letter-by-letter reading with shorter words easier or palm tracing (using tactile cues to imprint traced letters on the palm of hand). - May benefit from brief exposure to single words with repeated reading aloud
Hemianopic	- Homonymous hemianopia, often macular-splitting, often postgeniculate	- Slow but accurate text reading - May miss prefix or suffix - Left-sided more disabling than when in right visual fields
Neglect	- Right parietal lobe	- Errors on prefixes more frequent than on suffixes
Attentional	- Left parietal lobe	- Words merged - Letter crowding - Reads better with isolated words

make substitutions of one word for another word, although semantically related (i.e., table for chair). In that situation, there is a disturbance in sublexical and lexical processes required for spelling.

Lexical agraphia, also known as surface agraphia, is a written impairment in which the person over-relies on sound-to-letter conversions. Words with irregular spellings are often written as they sound ("right" written as "rit"). Phonological agraphia is the term used to describe the impairment experienced by a person who cannot write nonwords (for example, "prask") due to sublexical sound-to-letter conversion problems. People with phonological agraphia can write familiar words. Surface agraphia is another term used to describe an acquired writing impairment whereby the person reads by converting each letter to a sound so that irregularly spelled words are not pronounced correctly. For example,

the word "know" may be read with the /k/ audible. Those with surface agraphia can spell regular and nonsense words using phoneme-to-graphemes conversion but they misspell irregular words and homophones, for example, "sweet" and "suite." Barriere (2002) indicated in most people with aphasia, writing is the most impaired language function. Most often, patients with Broca's aphasia or a ranscortical motor aphasia have nonfluent agraphia and difficulty spelling (Duffy & Ulrich, 1976). Patients who do not have aphasia but have agraphia and alexia usually have parietal lobe lesions (Roeltgen, 1997).

Various treatment approaches can be found in Barriere (2002). One example is that of Beeson, Rewega, Vail, and Rapcsak (2000). The goal to help the patients problem-solve their spelling errors. In their research with patients who had spelling difficulties with a mild anomia, they taught them to use plausible misspellings gathered from sound-to-letter conversions. After writing words as they sounded, the task was to teach to patients to carefully monitor and self-correct spelling errors by considering their knowledge of the lexicon. They used an electronic speller that was able to accept plausible misspell-ings. Another treatment approach for individuals with Wernicke's aphasia and deficits at the level of graphemic output is the Anagram, Copy, and Recall Treatment (Beeson, 1999). This strategy, teaching patients to arrange anagram letters followed by repeated copying of words, has been successful.

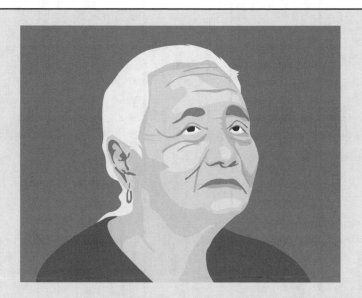

Case Scenario: Sue

History and Physical (H & P): 69-year-old, right-handed, Asian female, referred for outpatient cognitive-linguistic therapy 6 months s/p (status post), fell while shoveling snow; patient suffered a left hemispheric stoke in the distribution area of the posterior cerebral artery.

Past Medical History (PMH): HTN (hypertension), Diabetes Mellitus Type II, hypercholesterolemia; family history of cardiac problems.

Social History: Divorced; no children; lives alone w/ 2 cats; worked p/t as a teacher's aid in a local elementary school. Pt. upset about inability to work with children reading at school. ADLs (activities of daily living) are within normal limits (WNL).

Surgical History: Unremarkable.

A Functional Analysis of Sue's Alexia

Sue's reading skills are significantly impaired and should be the focus of her therapy. The therapist will need to decide if her approach will be restitutive or substitutive based on the residual reading that Sue still possesses. She is unable to participate in her favorite avocation—reading. Combining therapy for her word

Category	Assessment Area	Finding
Language Expression	Automatic Speech:	WFL for counting, reciting the alphabet, stating days and months of the year.
	Repetition Ability:	Repeating phrases and sentences are WFL.
	Lexical Retrieval-Naming:	Able to retrieve words with relative ease in discourse, however confrontation naming is a problem.
	Conversational Ability:	Syntax is WNL.
	Pragmatic Skills:	All social language skills WFL.
	Paraphasias:	None.
Speech	Rate:	WFL when not reading.
	Intelligibility:	WFL when not reading.
	Prosody:	WFL for inflection, rhythm, and stress of speech during conversation.
	Articulation:	WFL when not reading.
	Fluency:	WFL; average phrase length is 8+ words. Fluent speech output with ability to self-correct.
Auditory Comprehension	Answering Yes/No Questions:	WFL
	Executing Commands:	WFL
	Understanding Stories & Paragraphs:	WFL
	Understanding Conversational Speech:	Comprehension for words and sentences is intact. Can engage in conversational dialogue with minimal difficulty.
	Identifying Objects & their Functions:	WFL
Reading	Word-level Comprehension:	Compromised with difficulty processing word forms as a whole unit. Slow and inaccurate reading attempted with moderate-severe difficulty reading words. Short, common, and concrete words may be understood.
	Sentence-level Comprehension:	Impaired due to the reliance on sounding out words letter by letter. To facilitate rereading.
	Oral Reading:	Present difficulty reading aloud especially with irregularly spelled words, abstract words, and at the sentence level. Inaccurate pronunciation of those words attempted. Slow and labored. Some residual whole-word reading retained.
	Oral Spelling:	WFL for spelling concrete regularly spelled words' often relies on spelling letters to read words.
Written Expression	Copying:	WFL
	Writing to Dictation:	WFL
	Self-generated:	Writing is unaffected. Performs at same level prior to illness. Can write letters and take notes as necessary.
	Written Spelling:	WFL for regularly spelled words.
	Drawing:	WFL
Cognition	Alertness:	WFL
	Attention/Concentration:	WFL
	Visuospatial Skills:	WFL
	Memory:	WFL
	Executive Functions:	WFL
Behavioral Symptoms	Deficit awareness:	Aware of reading difficulty and attempts to improve daily using closed-caption television at home.
	Frustration:	Frustrated with inability to return to work as a teacher's aid.
	Emotional Lability:	None.
	Current Personality Characteristics:	Frustrated, angry and sad.

Figure 5–6. Diagnostic profile for Sue.

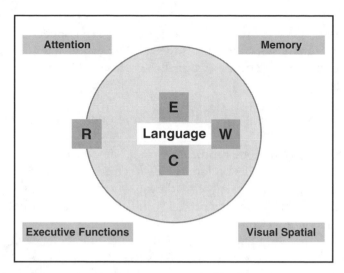

Figure 5–7. ALD Target Model for Sue.

retrieval problem with therapy for her alexia would be efficient. Furthermore, the "natural" relationship between writing/reading/naming will facilitate growth in each. The therapist will have to deal with Sue's frustration and anger over her impairment, especially as reading held such a prominent place in her life. Consequently, the therapist may want to point out the small successes that Sue makes, counseling her that these "building blocks" are crucial for any restitution of her reading ability. Sue's cognitive abilities are within functional limits which allow her to understand the implications of her deficits. This is advantageous from a treatment perspective.

Critical Thinking/Learning Activity

- What information indicates that this is a person with a pure alexia?
- How will Sue's reading problems affect her activities of daily living?
- What are the family counseling and education issues in this case, and how would you address them?
- Prepare a script reflecting a conversation between you and a caregiver who is trying to understand the complexity of Sue's reading problem.
- Write a SOAP note on this patient. Assume that you are seeing her for the first time after the evaluation session. Include three of the Short-Term Therapeutic Objectives in your note.

Treatment Considerations

Sue demonstrates functional receptive and expressive verbal language abilities. She is able to communicate effectively with her friends, watch TV with comprehension, and engage in normal phone conversations. Her speech is intelligible in all known and unknown contexts. However, her alexia has had a significant impact on her ability to return to work at the school and enjoy her favorite pastime: reading.

- There are two general types of treatment for alexia—*restitutive* and *substitutive*.
  - Restitutive Treatment approaches are designed to restore the impaired ability to its premorbid level. This is done by facilitating the underlying processes of reading.
    1. Present written words on cards and present them rapidly to discourage letter-by-letter reading.
    2. Use any method and materials that force the patient into relying on the residual whole-word skills that they may have.
  - Substitutive Treatment approaches are designed to compensate for the absent reading skills.
    1. Allow the patient to write the letter as she reads it, that is, use a kinesthetic modality to support the oral reading.
    2. Use any multimodality approach—tactile, tactile-kinesthetic, and visual—that can support the patient's reading of a letter or word.

Some Therapeutic Options

- Consider using the Anagram Copy and Recall Treatment (ACRT) (Beeson, 1999).
- Successful blending in a phonological reading treatment for deep alexia (Friedman & Lott, 2002).
- Computer-provided reading treatments (Katz & Wertz, 1997).
- ORLA VT (Oral Reading for Language in Aphasia with Virtual Therapist). (Cherney et al., 2005).

- Alexia Treatments in Perspectives on Neurophysiology and Neurogenic Speech and Language Disorders (Greenwald & George, 2002).

References

Barriere, I. (2002). Agraphia. *Perspectives on Neurophsyiology and Neurogenic Speech and Language Disorders, 12*(1), 13–20.

Beeson, P. (1999). Treating acquired writing impairment: Strengthening graphemic representations. *Aphasiology, 13*, 767–785.

Beeson, P. M., & Hillis, A. E. (2001). Comprehension and production of written words. In R. Chapey (Ed.), *Language intervention strategies in aphasia and related neurogenic communication disorders* (4th ed., pp. 572–604). Philadelphia: Lippincott Williams & Wilkins.

Beeson, P. M., Rewega, M., Vail, S., & Rapcsak, S. (2000). Problem-solving approach to agraphia treatment:

Interactive uses of lexical and sublexical spelling routes. *Aphasiology, 14*, 551-565.

Chapey, R. (2001). *Language intervention strategies in aphasia and related neurogenic communication disorders.* Philadelphia: Lippincott Williams & Wilkins.

Cherney, L. R., Babbitt, E. M., Cole, R., Van Vuuren, S., Hurwitz, R., Lee, J., et al. (2005). Oral reading for language in aphasia with virtual therapist. *The Center for Spoken Language Research (CSLR).* Retrieved December 6, 2007, from http://clear.colorado.edu/start/orla/orla.html

Duffy, F. H., & Geschwind, N. (1985). *Dyslexia: A neuroscientific approach to clinical evaluation.* Boston: Little, Brown & Company.

Duffy, R., & Ulrich, S. (1976). A comparison of impairments in verbal comprehension in speech, reading and writing in adult aphasics. *Journal of Speech and Hearing Disorders, 4*, 110-119.

Friedman, R., & Lott, N. (2002). Successful blending in a phonological reading treatment for deep aphasia. *Aphasiology, 16*(3), 355-372.

Greenwald, M., & George, P. (2002). Alexia. *Perspectives on Neurophsyiology and Neurogenic Speech and Language Disorders, 12*(1), 4-13.

Iragui, V. J., & Kritchevsky, M. (1991). Alexia without agraphia or hemianopia in parietal infarction. *Journal of Neurology, Neurosurgery, and Psychiatry, 54*, 841-842.

Katz, R., & Wertz, R. (1997). The efficacy of computer-provided reading treatment for chronic aphasic adults. *Journal of Speech, Language, and Hearing Research, 40*, 493-507.

Roeltgen, D. P. (1997). Agraphia. In T. E. Feinberg & M. J. Farah (Eds.), *Behavioral neurology and neuropsychology.* New York: McGraw-Hill.

Sinn, H., & Blanken, G. (1999). Visual errors in acquired dyslexia: Evidence for cascaded lexical processing. *Cognitive Neuropsychology, 16*, 631-653.

Chapter 6
RIGHT HEMISPHERE DISORDER

Characteristics

Individuals with right hemisphere disorder (RHD) typically do not have language problems as seen in those with aphasia. In a retrospective study, Blake et al. (2002) reviewed the medical charts of 123 patients who were admitted to an inpatient rehabilitation unit for RHD and found that only 45% were referred for speech-language pathology services, despite the fact that they presented with treatable communication and cognitive deficits. This suggests that referrals for speech-language pathology services are inadequate and underused in this clinical population.

The etiology of right hemisphere disorder (RHD) can be stroke, trauma, tumor, or degenerative disease and damage to the right cortical and subcortical structures is more diffuse than with left hemispheric damage. The consequence of this is more widespread dysfunction. The right hemisphere does not have a purely linguistic function, that is, it is not the seat of linguistic function, and therefore there is no aphasia present. However, it is now well established that unilateral damage to the right hemisphere can cause extralinguistic and paralinguistic deficits, which then produce communication impairment. *Extralinguistic impairments* include poor attentional skills, memory deficits, and visual-spatial difficulties. *Paralinguistic impairments* include pragmatic abnormalities; incohesive discourse, and tangential and circumlocutionary verbal output. It can be seen that a patient with a clinical presentation that includes these types of deficits will have problems in social discourse on a daily basis. Furthermore, these extra-linguistic and paralinguistic impairments can affect the patient's ability to be adequately assessed and consequently, produce an inconclusive or incorrect language picture. Thus, the clinician must be alert to the presence of these features during the assessment.

Not all patients will present with the same communicative characteristics (Tompkins & Fassbinder, 2004) and this causes problems for experimental design, data analysis, and combined with small sample sizes, affects the value of the results. Therefore, obtaining a valid representation of the communication disorder associated with right hemisphere brain damage has been challenging. Despite this, research has been able to provide the clinician with both verbal and nonverbal findings applicable to this population.

The patient with a right hemisphere disorder presents with perceptual, cognitive, and emotional deficits. Interpretation of linguistic and nonlinguistic information is problematic as they do not readily use context clues and have difficulty identifying what is important information in a communicative event from that which is unimportant. Following conversational rules is difficult and their speech can sound robotic due to an inability to vary prosody to reflect their emotional state at the time. Judgment and problem-solving abilities are also challenged. Nonlinguistic deficits are a hallmark in RHD. These patients may be disoriented to time and place, and have visuospatial deficits such as a left-sided neglect. Further complicating matters, the majority of RHD patients fail to recognize their own deficits (anosagnosia). In many cases the patient with RHD does not fully understand the extent of their disorder.

Communication Deficits

The following list comprises deficits commonly associated with RHD:

- Difficulty organizing information
- Impaired discourse
- Difficulty summarizing information in a meaningful way
- Impulsivity in their responses
- Tangential and circumlocutionary speech
- Using unnecessary detail in verbal communication
- Difficulty deciding what is relevant versus what is irrelevant to the context of the communicative event
- Difficulty using contextual cues
- Literal interpretation of idioms and indirect requests
- Pragmatic deficits, for example, speaker's intentions, understanding other's motivation, and following conventions of conversation.
- Reduced sensitivity to facial expression, gestures, body language, and the emotional content within verbal language,
- Difficulty understanding inferences based on context clues.

Visual-Perceptual Deficits

The person with a right hemisphere syndrome can present with an array of visual-perceptual impairments. *Visual agnosias* can manifest as an inability to recognize objects or colors. The patient will see and even handle an object, for example, a blue cup, yet not be able to tell what it is. This can have a very significant impact on the patient's ADLs. *Prosopagnosia* is defined as the inability to recognize faces, regardless of how familiar those faces are. Here again, one can see the devastating effects that this type of problem can have on the patient and his caregivers. Furthermore, this type of patient may also be unable to read facial expressions, for example, happy, sad, surprised, or angry. Difficulty with visual imagery can also have serious social conse-

quences. *Simultagnosia* is a disorder in which the patient cannot process the entire visual scene before him, but only attends to one part of the whole. Thus, the person misses the meaning of the image before him. *Visual integration deficits* are also observed with this population. Patients with this disorder are unable to form a cohesive visual percept from the stimuli before them. The visual image is not processed as integrated whole but rather as separate pieces. This problem along with *spatial disorientation* can affect the patient's ability to move around in space safely and efficiently.

Visuomotor Deficits

Associated with visual-perceptual problems are *visuomotor deficits*. The RHD patient may have difficulty dressing himself or herself as she is unable to orient her body to the placement of the clothing during dressing. From a diagnostic perspective, the patient will not be able to produce an accurate and correct clock drawing, and will be unable to construct objects in space, for example, build a tower of blocks or draw to express her needs. Both the drawings and the constructions will be inaccurate indicating to the clinician that there is a visuomotor deficit present.

Auditory Perceptual Deficits

Although auditory perceptual deficits are more often observed with bilateral lesions, it is possible that the RHD patient will present with some type of auditory perceptual difficulty. *Sound localization* difficulty may be observed as well as *auditory agnosia*, that is, an inability to "hone in" on the source of the auditory signal in space and the inability to recognize the sound as something familiar and/or meaningful. These patients also demonstrate problems with *discriminating prosodic patterns*, similar to the way that they are unable to discriminate facial expressions to convey meaning. The inability to perceive music appropriately is also a feature associated with RHD patients and this may be a factor in the functional life of a patient.

Cognitive Deficits

Attentional problems are very prevalent in this population. In order to sustain a dyadic communication, both partners must be attentive to the speech signal of the other. If the attention of one partner falters, then the probability that a successful communicative event will occur drops significantly. Furthermore, many patients with RHD present with left-sided neglect, or just an inattention to the left side. This can complicate the existing attentional problem since the patient is not able to make eye contact with the communication partner, unless he or she is on the patient's right side. A thorough chart review and diagnostic evaluation will highlight either of these issues for the speech-language pathologist.

The RHD patient may present with both *working memory* and *long-term memory* problems. Working memory is critical to functional language processing and long-term memory is necessary in order to access past knowledge and events. Deficits in both of these areas, although not directly related to speech and language, will affect the patient's ability to participate in social communication.

Clinicians working with RHD patients find that executive functioning is noticeably impaired. The neurophysiologic correlates to the relationship between the right hemisphere and executive functioning is most commonly seen in these patients are *planning difficulties*, impaired *problem-solving skills*, and difficulty *integrating* information. The role of attention in all of these functions is a critical element to performing them successfully and as noted above, these patients have significant attentional problems (Patterson & Chapey, 2008).

As noted above, there are several nonlinguistic deficits that often are encountered in persons with RHD. These primarily include left neglect, arousal deficits, and attention deficits including selective attention, more pronounced in the acute phase of the stroke. Myers (1998) reports that there tends to be less orientation to the environment in general. These patients also tend to have slower reaction times to both visual and auditory input and, in general, more intense stimulation is needed to facilitate attention than in a normally functioning individual. Because RHD patients tend to have reduced performance accuracy over time, attention for tasks is best when it is shorter in duration (Bub, Audet, & Lecours, 1990).

Research indicates that if distracters are present, the person with RDH exhibits slower performance and less accuracy in their responses. Neglect also increases when greater attention is required to complete a task (Kaplan, Verfailllie, Meadows, Caplan, Peasin, & de Witt, 1991).

Another performance deficit of RHD is the patient's difficulty integrating components into a whole. For example, the individual may draw a tire above the car instead of under the car indicating that they understand the components but have difficulty organizing them together into a coherent unit. Difficulty integrating and organizing information may also impact the patient's ability to express himself clearly in narrative form. These patients also tend to be tangential in their expressions, likely due to their difficulty staying on topic and getting to the point (Chapey, 2001).

Finally, it is worth mentioning that these paralinguistic and extralinguistic deficits are also associated with emotional factors. The clinician will note very soon after meeting an RHD patient that there is a flat facial affect, mirrored by a flat emotional affect. They have difficulty conveying emotions, and consequently appear distant and remote. These patients also have an impaired ability to process and produce appropriate prosodic patterns as well as facial expressions which further complicate their social interactions poststroke.

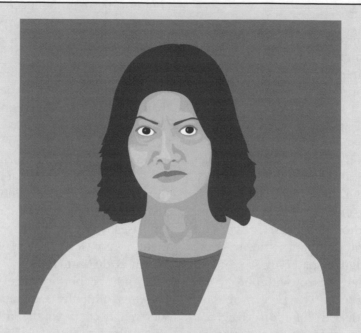

Case Scenario: Debra

History and Physical (H & P): 37-year old Latina female, right-handed, admitted via Emergency Department with twitching of the left hand and left upper extremity weakness. A CT scan revealed an infarct in the right frontal area, highly suggestive of a cerebrovascular accident. Family reported seizure-like movements × 1 at bedtime. Left-sided hemiparesis was also noted; left neglect noted.

Past Medical History (PMH): Right partial thyroidectomy, insomnia, chronic bronchitis; difficulty with gait, urinary incontinence.

Social History: Married; one child (21 months old); Ph.D. professor at a local university

Surgical History: s/p Thyroidectomy for a benign neoplasm.

A Functional Analysis of Debra's RHD

Debra's primary deficit areas are extralinguistic, prosodic, and cognitive. She is unable to process facial expressions, gestures, and body language. This interferes with her functional communication as nuanced meanings are missed, making her interpretations of the message very concrete and literal. Furthermore, she cannot accurately determine the speaker's intentions, which can easily produce misinterpretations. As Debra also has a left-sided neglect, she will not attend to people and/or objects located on her left side. Communication partners who are not aware that Debra has a left-sided neglect may feel as though Debra is ignoring them. Debra is also very dysprosodic making her sound robotic. Therefore, one aspect of her therapy must focus on developing proper pitch variations.

Figure 6–1. Diagnostic profile for Debra.

Language Expression
- Automatic Speech: WFL; able to count to 20, recite the alphabet, and name days and months of the year.
- Repetition Ability: WFL; difficulty noted with lengthy sentences (may be related to attentional deficit)
- Lexical Retrieval-Naming: WFL for confrontation naming and in conversation.
- Conversational Ability: Verbose, disorganized conversation with tangential and circumlocutionary output. Syntax WFL.
- Pragmatic Skills: Inappropriate turn-taking noted; her tangential output affects listener's attention.
- Paraphasias: None.

Speech
- Rate: Slow.
- Intelligibility: Good at conversational level in both known and unknown contexts.
- Prosody: Poor; flattened intonation with reduced stress patterns.
- Articulation: Mild consonantal distortions noted.
- Fluency: WFL

Auditory Comprehension
- Answering Yes/No Questions: WFL for simple and abstract questions.
- Executing Commands: WFL
- Understanding Stories & Paragraphs: WFL at word, phrase and sentence levels.
- Understanding Conversational Speech: Affected by inattentiveness.
- Identifying Objects & their Functions: WFL

Reading
- Word-level Comprehension: WFL
- Sentence-level Comprehension: Functional at the sentence and paragraph levels. However, unable to state the central theme of a complex paragraph.
- Oral Reading: WFL for monosyllabic and multisyllabic words; however errors noted at sentence level due to neglect and inattentiveness.
- Oral Spelling: WFL for monosyllabic and multisyllabic words.

Written Expression
- Copying: WFL
- Writing to Dictation: WFL for words and sentences.
- Self-generated: Writing functional sentences and notes WFL.
- Written Spelling: WFL for words and sentences.
- Drawing: WFL for simple line drawings.

Cognition
- Attention/Concentration: Poor; attention deteriorates with fatigue.
- Visuospatial Skills: Left neglect noted.
- Memory: Episodic memory, procedural memory, and semantic memory all WFL.
- Executive Functions: Difficulty with verbal problem-solving due to tangential output.

Behavioral Symptoms
- Alertness: WFL when well-rested.
- Deficit awareness: No awareness of deficits (anosagnosia).
- Frustration: Impatient and impulsive with noticeable frustration if listener offers corrections.
- Emotional Lability: None.
- Current Personality Characteristics: Depressed; lacks motivation; impulsive with her responses.

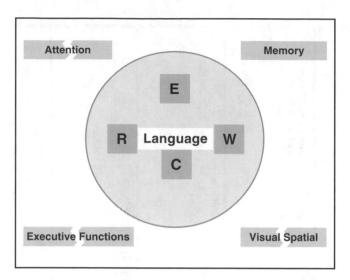

Figure 6–2. ALD Target Model for Debra.

This lack of appropriate intonation contours combined with Debra's flat affect make her a very challenging communication partner.

Her therapy also should focus directly on attention and neglect as well as the affective and prosodic components of communication. The goals for Debra would be to increase appropriate content in her communication; to improve her inferential abilities so she can make meaning of more than just the facts; and to facilitate her ability to generate meaning given ADL scenarios. For example, if a visitor walks into Debra's room and does not immediately greet her, she may not be able to correctly interpret that person's intentions, that is, she may believe that the visitor is angry with her. Therefore, helping Debra to develop alternate possibilities for people's behavior may assist her return to the social fabric of life. As noted above, Debra's inferential skills are weak and she has difficulty connecting an outcome to previous sequential events. For example, if you tell her that you went outside and then you came back in and were wet, one would infer that it was raining outside. However, Debra may not be able to make that inference and would need some facilitation in order to understand the inferential process. Also, reviewing the steps involved in completing a task verbally and in writing and then discussing the sequence prior to attempting the task may help facilitate functional problem-solving for ADL needs. For example, rehearsing and writing out the sequence of steps involved in a common household task, for example, making coffee or preparing a meal will be helpful. Similar scenarios, increasing in complexity and length, would be appropriate.

Cognitively, Debra has difficulty attending to stimuli and maintaining her focus. She is distractible and impulsive in her responses, and this is further complicated by fatigue. Visuospatial skills are compromised due to left visual neglect. Finally, Debra also presents with impairment in problem-solving and this is partially due to tangential thinking. Her episodic procedural and semantic memory systems are within functional limits (WFL) for activities of daily living (ADL) needs.

Critical Thinking/Learning Activity

- What information indicates that this patient has Right Hemisphere Dysfunction?
- This patient would most likely be seen in acute rehabilitation and then for outpatient therapy. Knowing that the insurance carrier will give you a limited number of sessions, how would you prioritize this patient's functional outcomes?
- What are the family counseling and education issues in this case, and how would you address them?
- How would you include the family/caregivers in this patient's treatment plan?
- Write a SOAP note on this patient. Assume that you are seeing her for the first time after the evaluation session. Include three short-term therapeutic objectives in your note.

Treatment Considerations

Debra is a functional communicator. She can carry on a conversation, however her flat affect and reduced intonation contours interfere with the social interaction during the communication event. Consequently, Debra appears disinterested and distracted during conversation. Although she is 100% intelligible in known and unknown contexts, Debra's speech is still characterized by articulatory distortions and a slow rate. Her voice is breathy and therefore she can be difficult to hear. Therefore, treatment must focus on the paralinguistic and extralinguistic aspects of her communication disorder as well as her speech production.

- Use contrastive stress drills with visual support to represent rising and/or falling intonation patterns. For example, in the sentence *I want to eat*, Debra must accent the appropriate word to respond to a wh-question such as "*Who* wants to eat?" Or "*What* do you want to do?" These provide Debra with a graphic representation of the intonation contour to facilitate her accurate production. Model as necessary.
- Increase loudness by providing visual feedback in the form of a sound level meter placed within Debra's view.
- Increase focus and attention use trail-making tasks and/or mazes. These tasks involve connecting letters or numbers in sequence across a page using a pencil.
- Improve Debra's ability to locate the left margin of a newspaper or magazine article by having her find the highlighted left margin, for example, a thick yellow line drawn down the left side of the page.

Some Therapeutic Options

■ Motoric-imitative treatment and cognitive-linguistic treatment (Rosenbek, Crucian, Leon, Hieber, Rodriguez, & Holiway, 2004; and Leon, Rosenbek, Crucian, Hieber, Holiway, & Rodriguez, 2005). The treatments have been based on theories that aprosodia is caused by motor programming deficits and a reduction in the ability to access emotionally charged words with prosody.

■ Psychoeducationally Based Program (Klonoff, Sheperd, O'Brien, Chiapello, & Hodak, 1990) investigated the appropriate use of context in pragmatics and discourse. Problems understanding discourse are often due to the abstract, nonliteral aspects of information. The program attempts to enhance independence through individual and group treatment focusing on emotional issues and pragmatics. Cognitive flexibility and visuospatial problem-solving are also reinforced.

■ Group Sessions focusing on Debra's attentional and affectual deficits.

■ Dysarthria therapy focusing on increasing loudness, articulatory distortions, and rate of speech.

■ Task-oriented treatments: these treatment approaches provide the patient with compensatory techniques useful for achieving a functional goal.

■ Process-oriented treatments: these treatment approaches optimize functional skills by working on the building blocks of those skills, that is, working on the parts of a skill and build the patient's skill set toward the whole.

References

Blake, M. L. (2007). Perspectives on treatment for communication deficits associated with right hemisphere brain damage. *American Journal of Speech-Language Pathology, 16*, 331–342.

Blake, M. L., Duffy, J. R., Myers, P. S., & Tompkins, C. A. (2002). Prevalence and patterns of right hemisphere cognitive communicative deficits: Retrospective data from an inpatient rehabilitation unit. *Aphasiology, 16*, 537–548.

Bub, D., Audet, T., & Lecours, A. R. (1990). Re-evaluating the effect of unilateral brain damage on simple reaction time to auditory stimulation. *Cortex, 26*, 227–237.

Kaplan, R. F., Verfaillie, M., Meadows, M. E., Caplan, L. R., Peasin, M. S., & deWitt, L. D. (1991). Changing attentional demands in left hemispatial neglect. *Archives of Neurology, 48*, 1263–1266.

Klonoff, P. S., Sheperd, J. C., O'Brien, K. P., Chiapello, D. A., & Hodak, J. A. (1990). Rehabilitation and outcome of right-hemisphere stroke patients: Challenges to traditional diagnostic and treatment methods. *Neuropsychology, 4*, 147–163.

Leon, S. A., Rosenbek, J. C., Crucian, G. P., Hieber, B., Holiway, B., & Rodriguez, A. D. (2005). Active treatments for aprosodia secondary to right hemisphere stroke. *Journal of Rehabilitation Research and Development, 42*, 93–102.

Myers, P. S. (1998). *Right hemisphere damage: Disorders of communication and cognition.* San Diego, CA: Singular.

Patterson, J. P., & Chapey, R. (2008). Assessment of language disorders in adults. In R. Chapey (Ed.), *Language intervention strategies in aphasia and related neurogenic communication disorders* (5th ed., pp. 64–160). Philadelphia: Wolters Kluwer/ Lippinsott Williams & Wilkins.

Rosenbek, J. C., Crucian, G. P., Leon, S. A., Hieber, B., Rodriguez, A. D., & Holiway, B. (2004). Novel treatments for expressive aprosodia: A phase I investigation of cognitive linguistic and imitative interventions. *Journal of the International Neuropsyuchological Society, 10,* 786-793.

Tompkins, C. A., & Fassbinder, W. (2004). Right hemisphere language disorders. In R. D. Kent (Ed.), *The MIT encyclopedia of communication disorders* (pp. 388-392). Cambridge, MA: MIT Press.

Chapter 7

TRAUMATIC BRAIN INJURY

Characteristics

Traumatic brain injury (TBI) is caused by a closed head injury, a penetrating head injury, or a deceleration injury which disrupt the normal functioning of the brain. The severity of TBI is very variable, and it can range from mild, with a brief change in consciousness and mental ability, to severe with coma and/or amnesia. In some cases, long-term disability results and the person is not able to return to his/her pre-morbid lifestyle. The risk of TBI is higher for men and for people between 0 to 4 years of age and 15 to 19 years old (Webb & Adler, 2008). Langlois, Rutland-Brown, and Thomas (2006) provide the more detailed statistics regarding incidence of TBI in the United States:

- In the United States, 1.4 million people sustain a TBI annually.
- Of the 1.4 million injured,
  - approximately 50,000 die
  - 235,000 are hospitalized
  - 1.1 million are treated in an emergency department and released.
- Approximately 475,000 cases of traumatic brain injuries occur among infants, children, and people under 14 years old.
- Adults who are 75 years and older have a higher hospitalization and mortality rate.
- The rate of head injury among males is twice that of females.

Individuals with TBI often present with a wide range of symptoms and disabilities. There is a phys-iologic disruption of brain functioning immediately following a traumatic brain injury. Most patients will experience an altered state of consciousness at the time of the injury. Some patients will lapse into a coma immediately, while others may gradually evolve into that state of consciousness. The majority of patients experience loss of memory for the events directly before the injury (retrograde amnesia) or after it (anterograde amnesia). Depending on the level of severity of the brain injury, the patient also may sustain focal or diffuse neurologic deficits and/or cognitive-linguistic impairment. Agitation is very common in the head injured patient. It can begin at the scene of the accident as "combativeness" and continue throughout the stages of recovery. The primary mechanisms of injury leading to TBI are illustrated in (Figure 7–1).

Types of Brain Injury

Although any change in brain neurophysiology and/or structure can be considered "traumatic," the term traumatic brain injury is much more specific in reference. The three most common types of TBI are due to: open head injury, closed head injury, and deceleration injuries. Stroke, hypoxia, tumors, infections, and toxic/metabolic processes are not considered TBI in this context, despite the changes in brain functioning that ensue. Table 7–1 describes the three types of head injury most typically associated with TBI.

The term "coup injury" refers to the injury at the point of contact. For example, if one sustains a blow to the left side of the head and only the left

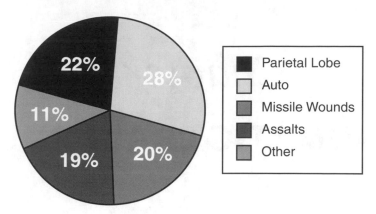

Figure 7–1. Primary mechanisms of injury causing TBI (Langlois, Rutland-Brown, & Thomas, 2006).

Table 7–1. Causes and Characteristics of TBI

Common Causes of TBI	Characteristics
Open Head Injury Example: Gunshot wound (GSW) to the head	Penetration of the skull (missile wound) with a direct injury to the brain. There is large focal damage and effects can be life-threatening. About 30 to 40% of patients experience seizures.
Closed Head Injury Examples: Assault with a blunt object; motor vehicle accident (MVA); falls	There is no penetration of the skull. Indirect force to the head is caused by rotation and/or deceleration. There is focal damage with the possibility of diffuse axonal injury. About 5% experience seizures. Coup and contrecoup injuries.
Deceleration Injuries Example: Head-on motor vehicle accident	Due to a sudden deceleration, the brain continues to move inside the skull as it moves at a different rate than the skull because it is soft. There tends to be diffuse axonal shearing, contusions, and brain swelling due to repeated back and forth motion inside the skull. If axons tear, the neurons die.

hemisphere is affected, then the patient has experienced a *coup injury*. If, however, the patient sustains damage in the right hemisphere after a blow to the left side of the head, then that is termed a *contrecoup injury*. Thus, these two lesion sites arise from the original blow to the brain (coup injury) and the other contusion is a result of the brain rebounding off the skull at the site opposite of impact (contrecoup injury). Shearing forces occur if there is a rapid and forceful motion of the head, which is often the case in auto accidents. For example, in an auto accident, the patient's brain still may be moving in an anterior-posterior direction after the car has stopped. Such movement can cause *diffuse axonal injury* due to tearing of axons and the myelin sheath covering them.

There is also a loss of consciousness accompanied by swelling (edema) of the brain and vascular damage deep within the brain. If pressure in the skull is not stopped through surgery, cooling, medication, or by other medical intervention, the brain will swell to the point that it is pushed down through the opening at the skull's base (the foramen magnum). This is referred to as *brain herniation*. Consequently, the brainstem nuclei controlling breathing and heart functions will be compressed and the person will die. Abnormal posturing may result from brain herniation and there are two types that can be observed in people with TBI: *decorticate posturing*, due to unilateral or bilateral corticospinal tract damage; or *decerebrate posturing* which indicates that there is swelling of the upper brainstem. The severity and duration of these abnormal postures contribute to the favorability of the patient's long-term outcome, that is, the longer the duration and the more severe the posturing then the poorer the long-term prognosis (Springhouse, 2007). Figure 7–2 illustrates the two types of abnormal posturing.

Prognostic Considerations in Head Injury

The clinician working with a patient who has TBI s/p head injury will need to consider five general variables in relation to functional outcome: premorbid intelligence, age at the time of injury, dura-

tion of coma, posttraumatic amnesia and medical complications during the hospital stay. There are other variables which also can impact functional outcome, such as gender and initial Glasgow Coma Scale (GCS) score (Brown et al., 2005), so if the clinician is attentive to all of these factors, a very reasonable prognostic picture for the patient can be formulated.

Premorbid Intelligence

Kesler et al. (2003) tested the concept of cognitive reserve in 24 patients with brain injury. Cognitive reserve has been postulated as the factor to explain the individual difference in functional outcomes. Using MRI imaging, the authors measured total intracranial volume and ventricle-to-brain ratio. They also looked at educational level and premorbid standardized testing and compared it with the subject's cognitive outcome postinjury. Their results found that

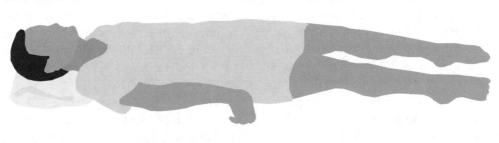

A. Extension posturing (decerebrate rigidity)

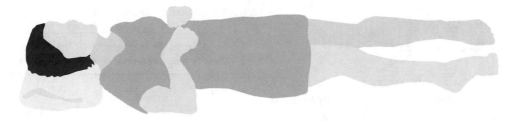

B. Abnormal flexion (decorticate rigidity)

Figure 7–2. Decerebrate and decorticate postures. (**A**) Extension posturing (decerebrate rigidity), and (**B**) Abnormal flexion (decorticate rigidity).

larger premorbid brain volume and higher education level may decrease vulnerability to cognitive deficits following TBI, consistent with the notion of a cognitive reserve.

Age at the Time of Injury

Age at the time of injury appears to be a strong indicator of morbidity and functional outcome Wetzel & Squire, 1982). If the patient is 40 years of age or under a good outcome is predicted in most cases. However, if the patient is over 50 the outcome is poorer and poorer still if the patient is over 60 years of age (Brain Trauma Foundation, 2000a).

Duration of Coma

There are two factors to consider in relation to coma: duration of coma and depth of coma. Duration is measured in weeks, and there appears to be a direct and linear relationship between recovery and the duration of the coma. Depth of coma is based on the GCS score. Patients whose coma lasts less than two weeks have better prognosis for full recovery than those whose coma lasts longer than two weeks (Brain Trauma Foundation, 2000b). When the patient is first encountered by medical professionals and the GCS is administered within 24 hours of the injury, those with a score less than 8 are a higher risk than those with a score greater than 8. If the GCS is administered 24 hours after the injury, a score of 5 or less indicates a poor outcome and greater than 5 is predictive of a good outcome (Brain Trauma Foundation, 2000b).

Posttraumatic Amnesia

Another prognosticator for recovery after head injury is the duration of amnesia. Typically, people who sustain head injury have no memory of the actual event. However, as they recover they may be able to "go back in time" and begin to remember events closer and closer to the actual incident. If the post-traumatic amnesia is less than two weeks prior to

patient's admission to the hospital then the prognosis for a fuller recovery is better than if it is greater that 12 weeks prior to admission. This is dependent on the severity of the injury, the type of injury and the communication skills of the patient. The clinician can monitor this amnesia which will help in prognostication and even therapy planning. Table 7–2 provides expectations for full recovery given the amount of time with post-traumatic amnesia.

Medical Complications

In order to obtain a rapid clinical picture of the patient, the first assessment tool used by medical professionals on their first encounter with the head injured patient is the Glasgow Coma Scale (GCS) (Jennett & Bond, 1975). This typically occurs in the field, that is, at the scene of the accident or injury, as the patient is being stabilized for transport. However, the GCS also can be administered by EMTs in the helicopter transporting the patient to the hospital, or in the emergency department upon arrival to the hospital. The patient is rated according to his eye opening response, verbal response, and motor response. These scores are then tallied and a score is obtained. The highest score obtainable on the GCS is 15. The lowest score obtainable is 3. Teasdale and Jennett (1974) describe a GCS score of 3 to 8 as severe TBI, 9 to 12 as moderate TBI, and 13 to 15 as mild TBI. It is important to remember that a patient may improve despite a low GCS score; however, it is generally held that a score between 8 and 15 repre-

Table 7–2. Relationship Between Duration of Post-Traumatic Amnesia and Recovery Time

Time of posttraumatic amnesia experienced	Time expected for full recovery
Less than 5 minutes	1 month
5 to 60 minutes	3 months
1–24 hours	1 year
1–7 days	1–2 years
8–28 days	Residual deficits remain

sents a more favorable diagnosis. Table 7–3 shows the rating scale of the GCS.

Dawodu (2007) further refines the criteria for severity of brain injury as follows:

- A diagnosis of mild brain injury is made when:
  - The GCS score greater than 12
  - There are no abnormalities noted on CT scan
  - There are no operative lesions
  - The length of stay in the hospital is less than 48 hours
- A diagnosis of moderate brain injury is made when:
  - GCS score of 9 to 12 or higher
  - Abnormal CT scan findings
  - Operative intracranial lesion
  - The length of stay in the hospital is at least 48 hours
- A diagnosis of severe brain injury is made when:
  - The GCS score is below 9 within 48 hours of the injury.

Medical complications after TBI are common and myriad. Of course, the level of severity of the initial head injury plays a role in the extent and nature of these problems, that is, the more severe the more likely those complications will arise post-injury. We briefly summarize below the medical complications that the speech-language pathologist will most likely encounter in the acute care and rehab phases of the patient's hospitalization: post-traumatic seizures, hydrocephalus, and spasticity.

Table 7–3. The Glasgow Coma Scale

Eye Opening Response	Spontaneous—open with blinking at baseline	4 points
	Opens to verbal command, speech, or shout	3 points
	Opens to pain, not applied to face	2 points
	None	1 point
Verbal Response	Oriented	5 points
	Confused conversation, but able to answer questions	4 points
	Inappropriate responses, words discernible	3 points
	Incomprehensible speech	2 points
	None	1 point
Motor Response	Obeys commands for movement	6 points
	Purposeful movement to painful stimulus	5 points
	Withdraws from pain	4 points
	Abnormal (spastic) flexion, decorticate posture	3 points
	Extensor (rigid) response, decerebrate posture	2 points
	None	1 point

Posttraumatic Seizures

Posttraumatic seizures (PTS) are a common complication of TBI and most commonly occur after moderate and severe head injury. Seizures are classified based on how soon after the initial injury they occur: immediate seizures occur within 24 hours of the injury, early seizures occur in the 2 to 7 days postinjury, and late seizures occur any time after day 7 postinjury (Pangilinan, 2008). Late onset posttraumatic seizures occur in 5 to 19% of those with brain injury and approximately one-third to half of all brain-injured patients develop them (Bushnik et al., 2004).

Hydrocephalus

The four ventricles of the brain comprise the ventricular system whose function is to keep the brain and spinal cord bathed in cerebral spinal fluid (CSF). The CSF circulates continuously and is reabsorbed back into the bloodstream. Hydrocephalus occurs when the CSF cannot exit the ventricles, builds up there, and causes significant pressure on the adjacent cortical areas. In TBI the two most common types of hydrocephalus are *communicating* and *noncommunicating*. If there is an obstruction in the subarachnoid space, preventing the free flow of CSF, communicating hydrocephalus results and this is the most common type found in TBI. An obstruction in the ventricular system that prevents the CSF from exiting the fourth ventricle results noncommunicating hydrocephalus (Parcell et al., 2006).

Spasticity

Elovic and Zafonte (2001) found that in one inpatient rehabilitation unit 25% of the patients demonstrated spasticity. Spasticity is a sign of upper motor neuron damage whereas rigidity is a sign of basal ganglia involvement. The important fact that the speech-language clinician must keep in mind is that some medications used to reduce spasticity and rigidity may cause cognitive deficits, especially the use of baclofen, tizanidine, clonidine, and benzodiazepines (Pangilinan, 2008).

Cognitive-Linguistic Impairment Due to TBI

There are three major deficit areas that result from TBI. These are neurologic/physical impairments, cognitive/intellectual impairments, and emotional/behavioral impairments. Neurologically, there may be coordination problems, epilepsy, paresis (unilateral or bilateral), sensory, and/or perceptual impairments, to name a few. Cognitive impairment also may arise and includes deficits of memory, intellectual quotient, processing speed, attention, executive functioning, and/or communication problems. Emotional and behavioral complications are very common in this population. The person may display personality changes, difficulty self-monitoring, a lack of motivation, impulsivity, aggression, disinhibition, anxiety, and/or depression, with limited awareness. Language deficits occur in one-third of severe TBI survivors but rarely evident in cases of mild TBI. Table 7–4 summarizes the deficit areas and offers some treatment considerations.

In children, outcomes are impacted by the severity of the TBI, the site and size of the lesion and age. Children with mild TBI generally make the most improvements within 6 months post injury whereas those with severe TBI and more diffuse damage tend to make gradual improvements over an 18 month postinjury time frame. Children with brain injury often recover more readily because the language areas are more flexible (plasticity). As they become older, the areas become more specialized and less resilient (Szaflarski, 2006).

Postconcussive Syndrome

Not all head injury produces significant TBI. Mild TBI is characterized by no loss of consciousness or one that lasts less than 20 minutes with a hospitalization that is less than 72 hours. The score on the GCS is greater than 12. *Postconcussive syndrome* (PCS) has been identified as a sequela to mild brain injury in some cases (Legome & Wu, 2006). Mild injury is characterized by a brief loss of consciousness and/or post-traumatic amnesia and may also

Table 7–4. Primary Deficits in TBI and Areas for Treatment

Primary Type of Deficits	Treatment Considerations
Cognitive-Communication	Word finding is a major deficit in severe TBI and can be seen in mild cases, though to a lesser degree of impairment. There is difficulty organizing and sequencing information. Speech is often tangential, and the patient is unable to differentiate relevant from irrelevant information when formulating a discourse. Expressing and comprehending humor can be impaired. Understanding of abstract language and expression is often limited. Synthesizing written information can also be impaired.
	Pragmatic language is often impaired, for example, eye contact, affect, use of gestures, and understanding of body language and facial expressions are deficient. Pragmatic deficits also include topic selection and maintenance, expression of complex ideas, and making inappropriate comments. Narrative discourse is incohesive. Automatic and overlearned language is often unaffected.
Academic	There is difficulty organizing, integrating, and generalizing information to another context. Self-awareness of problems is limited and there is poor planning ability. Self-monitoring of errors and behaviors are weak.
	An individual is often ready for school when they can attend to a task for 15–20 minutes and they can tolerate 20–30 minutes of stimulation. They should also be able to function in a group of 2 or more and engage in meaningful communication with the ability to follow basic directions. There should be an interest in learning.
Executive Functioning	Three areas must be considered: executing cognitive plans, managing time, and self-regulating. A fully functioning individual needs to possess the ability to organize and sequence plans and initiate activities to work toward goals. They also should work toward estimating time and creating schedules to carry out activities and change plans if needed. In order to self-regulate, the individual must judge their own behavior to complete tasks, control impulses, work without perseveration, and act independently.
Memory	During the sensory store stage, stimuli enter the system (visual, auditory, tactile, emotional, etc.) and disappear. Short-term working memory is limited and tends to last 20 seconds or less. It is assisted by rehearsal, visuospatial sketchpad, and decision-making. Long-term memory lasts from minutes to years. Consolidation must occur for this to work for later recall. Three memory systems, semantic knowledge, episodic or event-based, and procedural are important to communication.

demonstrate disorientation. Interestingly, more men sustain mild brain injury, but the incidence of PCS is higher in women. Fifty percent of mild brain injury patients are between the ages of 15 and 34. The PCS patient may also present with a Glasgow Coma Scale (GCS) of 13 to 15, and some even 15 (Legome & Wu, 2006). Legome & Wu (2006) also report that between 29 to 90% of patients will experience postconcussive symptoms after mild brain injury and these patients tend not to report to the ED immediately after the injury. Approximately 15% of PCS patients will continue to report problems 12 months after the injury, which may be refractory to treatment, leaving the patient with a lifelong disability (Legome & Wu, 2006).

The diagnosis of PCS remains controversial. However, Legome & Wu (2006) feels that if headache, dizziness, fatigue, irritability, impaired memory and concentration, insomnia, and lowered tolerance for noise and light continues after the injury, than the diagnosis can be made. He believes that PCS can at least be loosely defined as a persistence of these symptoms within several weeks after the initial insult. Kalinian (2008) states that PCS is a "cluster of cognitive, behavioral, and emotional symptoms that occur after a blow, a fall, or hit to the head" (p.1). The most common symptom of PCS are:

- Persistent low-grade headaches that linger
- Attentional difficulties or problems concentrating
- Difficulty remembering things
- Problems with planning and organization
- A new and noticeable "slowness" in thinking
- Disorientation resulting in getting lost more easily
- Reduced energy level
- Changes in the senses of smell and/or taste
- Tinnitus
- Changes in behavior and personality such as anxiety, depression, irritability, sleep abnormalities, changes in appetite, and changes in libido.

Diagnostic testing may identify weaknesses in the following areas:

- Vocabulary
- Short-term and immediate memory
- Attention
- Cognitive flexibility
- Information processing

- Object recall
- Drawing
- Mathematics

The clinician must be alert to those patients who experience very mild cognitive-linguistic impairment upon initial testing. He must present detailed prophylactic counseling and education to the caregivers regarding PCS. In the case of children, the clinician must consider giving a copy of the evaluation report to the child's teachers so that any special programming can be arranged. Follow-up cognitive-linguistic testing should also be considered approximately 6 weeks s/p discharge to monitor the trends in the recovery process and to rule out the emergence of any new impairments.

Rating Scales for Functional Outcomes

The GCS is designed to provide the first responders and the medical team with a clinical picture of the patient immediately after the injury and for the early stage of the hospitalization. It does not address the cognitive, linguistic, behavioral and functional outcomes as well as two other scales: The Rancho Los Amigos Level of Cognitive Functioning Scale (Northeast Center for Special Care, 2007; Hagen et al., 1972; Malkmus & Stenderup, 1974)[1] and the Disability Rating Scale (Rappaport et al., 1982). We review the scales and their function below.

The Rancho Los Amigos Scale (RLA)

Currently, there are 10 levels of function which are defined by the patient's behavior, including functional communication skills. The clinician uses the RLA during the initial assessment and for follow-up monitoring of the patient. In both the acute-care phase of the patient's recovery and in the rehabilitative phase, the RLA is useful for goal planning and

---

[1]Original Scale co-authored by Chris Hagen, Ph.D., Danese Malkmus, M.A., Patricia Durham, M.A. Communication Disorders Service, Rancho Los Amigos Hospital, 1972. Revised 11/15/74 by Danese Malkmus, M.A., and Kathryn Stenderup, O.T.R.

prognostication. Each level of the scale has more detailed behavioral and communication characteristics associated with it, but in the representation of the scale below, we have included only the general clinical presentation. We refer the reader to http://www.rancho.org/ which is the Web site of Ranchos Los Amigos National Rehabilitation Center for the fuller version of this scale. We recommend that the clinician continually monitor the patient's progress by using the scale at each bedside or office visit, starting with the initial evaluation session in the hospital. Table 7–5 describes the RLA.

The Disability Rating Scale (DRS)

The DRS (Rappaport et al., 1982), provides a very functional picture of the brain-injured patient to those around him (Table 7–6). Unlike the RLA, the DRS covers the full range of human activity that must be considered if full recovery is to be addressed. This scale can be used at the early stages of hospitalization through the community re-entry phase of recovery. Furthermore, the DRS is a perfect platform upon which to design interdisciplinary goals which would enhance the patient's functional outcome.

Table 7–5. The Ranchos Los Amigos Levels of Cognitive Function Scale (RLA) Showing the Levels of Cognitive Functioning and Behavioral Characteristic Associated with Each Level

Levels of Cognitive Functioning	Clinical Presentation
Level I	No Response: Total Assistance
Level II	Generalized Response: Total Assistance
Level III	Localized Response: Total Assistance
Level IV	Confused/Agitated: Maximal Assistance
Level V	Confused Inappropriate Nonagitated: Maximal Assistance
Level VI	Confused Appropriate: Moderate Assistance
Level VII	Appropriate: Minimal Assistance for Daily Living Skills
Level VIII	Purposeful Appropriate: Standby Assistance
Level IX	Purposeful Appropriate: Standby Assistance on Request
Level X	Purposeful Appropriate: Modified Independent

Table 7–6. The Disability Rating Scale (DRS)

Category	Item	Instructions	Score
Arousability, Awareness, and Responsivity	Eye Opening	0 = *spontaneous* 1 = *to speech* 2 = *to pain* 3 = *none*	
	Communication Ability	0 = *oriented* 1 = *confused* 2 = *inappropriate* 3 = *incomprehensible* 4 = *none*	
	Motor Response	0 = *obeying* 1 = *localizing* 2 = *withdrawing* 3 = *flexing* 4 = *extending* 5 = *none*	
Cognitive Ability for Self-Care Activities	Feeding	0 = *complete* 1 = *partial* 2 = *minimal* 3 = *none*	
	Toileting	0 = *complete* 1 = *partial* 2 = *minimal* 3 = *none*	
	Grooming	0 = *complete* 1 = *partial* 2 = *minimal* 3 = *none*	
Dependence on Others	Level of Functioning	0 = *completely independent* 1 = *independent in special environment* 2 = *mildly dependent* 3 = *moderately dependent* 4 = *markedly dependent* 5 = *totally dependent*	
Psychosocial Adaptability	Employability	0 = *not restricted* 1 = *selected jobs* 2 = *sheltered workshop (noncompetitive)* 3 = *not employable*	
		Total DRS Score	

Disability Categories: 0 (Total DR Score) = None (Level of Disability); 1 = Mild; 2–3 = Partial; 4–6 = Moderate; 7–11 = Moderately Severe; 12–16 = Severe; 17–21 = Extremely Severe; 22–24 = Vegetative State; 25–29 = Extreme Vegetative State.

Source: Reprinted with permission from: *Archives of Physical Medicine and Rehabilitation, 63*, Rappaport et al., Disability rating scale for severe head trauma patients: Coma to community, pp. 118–123. Copyright Elsevier (1982).

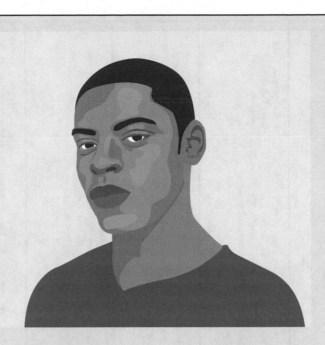

Case Scenario: Samuel

History and Physical (H & P): 22-year-old African American male admitted s/p motor vehicle accident (MVA) versus tree with lateral impact; patient was unrestrained and found partially ejected from the vehicle; combative but conscious on the scene; moving all extremities. Initial CT scan of the head revealed bilateral mandibular fractures and diffuse subarachnoid hemorrhage (SAH) at the vertex; subdural hematoma (SDH) at the falx; Glasgow Coma Scale (GCS) in ED: 9/15.

Past Medical History (PMH): No significant past medical history; independent with all ADLs prior to this admission.

Social History: Lives alone; high school graduate with a history of learning disability; works in environmental services for a local hospital.

Surgical History: Unremarkable.

A Functional Analysis of Samuel's TBI

Once Samuel is stabilized in the acute care phase of his recovery, most, if not all, of his rehabilitation will take place in a brain injury unit at a rehabilitation hospital. Typically, patients like Samuel will be discharged to a free-standing rehabilitation hospital for a short stay and then to home. He will then begin outpatient services including a community re-entry program. In order to return to work and his premorbid social environment, Samuel will need to improve both his communication skills and his behaviors, as deficits in both areas will affect his employability and his ability to establish and maintain social relationships. The clinician must always focus on the three major areas of impairment in people

Language Expression	**Automatic Speech:** WFL for counting, days of the week, alphabet with a verbal prompt to facilitate initiation.	**Repetition Ability:** WFL for words and sentences.	**Lexical Retrieval-Naming:** Confrontation naming is WFL when interested in participating.	**Conversational Ability:** Difficulty maintaining a conversational thread; however, he can respond to simple questions accurately.	**Pragmatic Skills:** Intermittent turn-taking errors; poor eye contact; flat affect; occasional taboo language noted in response to questioning; spontaneous utterances are WFL. / **Paraphasias:** None.
Speech	**Rate:** WFL	**Intelligibility:** WFL in known and unknown contexts; hypophonia can affect intelligibility.	**Prosody:** Monotone.	**Articulation:** WFL	**Fluency:** WFL
Auditory Comprehension	**Answering Yes/No Questions:** WFL for simple yes/no questions; perseveration noted on items of increased complexity.	**Executing Commands:** WFL for simple one-step commands.	**Understanding Stories & Paragraphs:** Poor auditory comprehension at the paragraph level; patient perseverated on a "yes" response to all questions related to the material in the paragraph.	**Understanding Conversational Speech:** Poor; has difficulty understanding connected speech.	**Identifying Objects & their Functions:** WFL
Reading	**Word-level Comprehension:** Mildly impaired, worse on multisyllabic and abstract words.	**Sentence-level Comprehension:** Moderately impaired; However, pre-morbidly patient read at the 4th – 5th grade level and was in learning support throughout high school.	**Oral Reading:** Reading aloud is slow and labored.		**Oral Spelling:** WFL for monosyllabic words; spelling polysyllabic words impaired and may be due to memory impairment (may be at pre-morbid level according to parent).
Written Expression	**Copying:** Copies basic shapes and letters when attentive.	**Writing to Dictation:** Unable to comply with directions.	**Self-generated:** Functional for name, but not his address; legible but disorganized.	**Written Spelling:** Poor at word level; may be due to pre-morbid learning disability complicated by current head injury.	**Drawing:** Scribbles when given pen and paper.
Cognition	**Attention/Concentration:** Externally distractible and resentful of re-direction to task. Selective attention is poor for tasks requiring sustained concentration.	**Visuospatial Skills:** WFL for ADL needs in hospital environment.	**Memory:** Short-term memory impaired for semantic and episodic information; better at procedural tasks. Long-term memory is mildly impaired for events from recent past. Retrograde amnesia present.	**Executive Functions:** Requires daily and frequent orientation to time/place/date. Poor problem solving for home-based ADLs; perseverated on "I don't know," and "That's a stupid question." Safety awareness is poor in all environments. Unable to sequence a series of daily events to plan his day.	
Behavioral Symptoms	**Alertness:** Variable, but improved from baseline on admission.	**Deficit awareness:** Poor; unaware of communication deficits; poor self-monitoring skills.	**Frustration:** Not noted at the time of assessment.	**Emotional Lability:** Periodic tearfulness observed during therapy sessions.	**Current Personality Characteristics:** Emotional outbursts are common; Flat affect; irritable.

Figure 7–3. Diagnostic profile for Samuel.

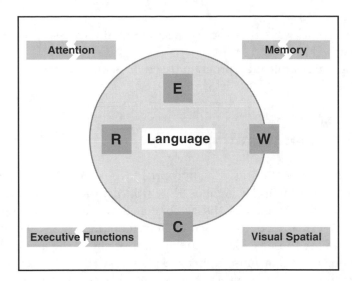

Figure 7–4. ALD Target Model for Samuel.

with TBI: the neurologic and physical, the cognitive-linguistic, and the behavioral/emotional. Not every patient will demonstrate equal impairment in all three areas. For example, Sam has cognitive-linguistic impairment as well as behavioral difficulties. Other patients may demonstrate significant cognitive-linguistic deficits yet have fewer behavioral challenges, although this is a rarer scenario in the context of significant cognitive-linguistic deficits.

Treatment for Samuel must address his cognitive deficits and his irritability. He will have more difficulty becoming a contributing member to society if he cannot solve problems, think critically, and have an insightful understanding of his deficit areas. Therefore, helping Samuel develop self-monitoring skills to prevent emotional outbursts is important. Here the SLP can cotreat with a rehabilitation psychologist and other professionals, each focusing on aspects within their own scope of practice. Or, the SLP can reinforce the self-monitoring techniques that the psychologist taught Samuel to use when necessary. Samuel's memory deficits must be addressed very early during his rehabilitation. Without a functional memory, Samuel will be dependent on others for certain ADLs. Finally, family counseling and education must always be an integral part of Samuel's rehabilitation program. The family will need support and information to help them manage and understand the "new Sam," as he charts a challenging course back to functional cognitive-linguistic and behavioral skills.

Critical Thinking/Learning Activity

1. What are some tools that you can use to monitor Samuel's auditory comprehension progress? How would you chart this data?
2. How will you manage Samuel's attentional problems during the evaluation?

3. What are some ways that you can use the family to assist you in Samuel's treatment?
4. Design a family education program based on Samuel's profile.
5. How will you use the DRS in Samuel's case?

Treatment Considerations

Samuel was at Level V (Confused Inappropriate Nonagitated, requiring maximal assistance) on the Rancho Los Amigos Scale (RLA) at the time of evaluation and his DRS score was 5 (Moderate). His lack of deficit awareness, impaired attention (poor eye contact), and compromised auditory comprehension will create challenges to his ability to participate in therapy, especially in the acute phase of his hospitalization. The team must immediately address Samuel's attentional problems so that he can participate in therapy and process incoming information. This is critical, especially during his acute care hospitalization, when many staff members are working with him and making requests of him so that they can help him. Daily monitoring of his attentional, executive functions and auditory processing skills is critical for planning the next level of care for Samuel. The RLA and the DRS would be useful in this regard. In the acute care phase of TBI, the major emphasis is on assessment and monitoring progress, for example, via the RLA, the DRS, and serial testing, so that the therapist at the next level of care have the information the need to establish optimal, realistic and function rehabilitation goals. The three primary areas that need to be addressed in this case in order to optimize Samuel's functional communication and prepare him for rehabilitation are:

- Auditory comprehension
- Behavior
- Executive functioning

The following are more detailed treatment considerations for Samuel's case:

- It is important to demonstrate patience. Samuel will need more time to process and respond. You also will need to be aware that as he moves through the Rancho levels, his behavior will become more manageable.
- Supplement auditorily presented information with pictures and words. This will optimize his response by engaging his visual attention system.
- Talk to nursing about the medications that Samuel is prescribed. This will affect his ability to participate and even determine the most optimal time for your session with him.
- Design auditory comprehension tasks that build on Samuel's strengths, for example, start at the one-step command level gradually building to more complexity.

- Reinforcing his successful trials will facilitate compliance and engagement in therapy.
- Use objects, sentences, tasks that relate to his current needs. For example, use his toothbrush and comb during a processing task instead of disconnected and abstract commands.
- Reinforce positive and compliant behavior during therapy. Use the reinforcement schedule that is most appropriate for his age and one which will ensure generalization of the desired behavior(s).
- Provide continual counseling and education to Samuel's caregivers. Engage them in the therapeutic process so that they can get firsthand knowledge about his skills and deficit areas. Teach them how to implement your program with Samuel.

Therapeutic Options

- Peer group training of pragmatic skills (Wiseman-Hakes, Stewart, Wasserman, & Schuller, 1998).
- Web-based family problem-solving intervention (Wade, Wolfe, Brown, & Pestian, 2005).
- Behavioral interventions for behavior disorders after TBI (Ylvisaker, Turkstra, Coelho, et al., 2007).
- Social skills intervention for adolescents with TBI (Turkstra & Burgess, 2007).
- Intervention for memory disorders after TBI (Avery & Kennedy, 2007).
- Treatment of discourse deficits following TBI (Cannizzaro, Coelho, & Youse, 2007).
- Teaching compensatory strategies: modeling, direct instruction, and functional practice (Ylvisaker, Szekeres, & Feeney, 2008).
- The Rivermead Postconcussion Symptoms Questionnaire (King, Crawford, & Wenden, et al., 1995).

References

Avery, J., & Kennedy, M. R. T. (2007). Intervention for memory disorders after TBI. *Traumatic brain injury: Cognitive communication rehabilitation* (pp. 10–15). Rockville, MD: ASHA.

Brain Trauma Foundation. (2000a, June). The American Association of Neurological Surgeons: The joint section on neurotrauma and critical care. *Journal of Neurotrauma, 17*(6–7), 573–581.

Brain Trauma Foundation. (2000b, June). The American Association of Neurological Surgeons: The joint section on neurotrauma and critical care. Glasgow Coma Scale score. *Journal of Neurotrauma, 17*(6–7), 563–571.

Brown, A. W., Malec, J. F., McClelland, R. L., Diehl, N. N., Englander, J., & Cifu, D. X. (2005). Clinical elements that predict outcome after traumatic brain injury: A prospective multicenter recursive partitioning (decision-tree) analysis. *Journal of Neurotrauma, 22*(10), 1040–1051.

Bushnik, T., Englander, J., & Duong, T. (2004). Medical and social issues related to posttraumatic seizures in persons with traumatic brain injury. *Journal of Head Trauma Rehabilitation, 19*(4), 296–304.

Cannizzaro, M. S., Coelho, C. A., & Youse, K. (2007). Treatment of discourse deficits following TBI. *Traumatic brain injury: Cognitive communication rehabilitation* (pp. 17–21). Rockville, MD: ASHA.

Dawodu, S. T. (2007). *Traumatic brain injury: Definition, epidemiology, and pathophysiology.* Retrieved September 6, 2008, from http://www.emedicine.com/pmr/TOPIC212.HTM

Elovic, E., & Zafonte, R. D. (2001). Spasticity management in traumatic brain injury. *Physical Medicine Rehabilitation State of Art Review, 15*, 327–348.

Jennett, B., & Bond, M. (1975). Assessment of outcome after severe brain damage. *Lancet, 1*, 480–484.

Kalinian, H. (2008). *Definition of Postconcussive syndrome or concussion.* Retrieved September 6, 2008, from http://www.neuropsychconsultant.com/postconcussive.html

Kesler, S. R., Adams, H. F., Blasey, C. M., & Bigler, E. D. (2003). Premorbid intellectual functioning, education, and brain size in traumatic brain injury: An investigation of the cognitive reserve hypothesis. *Applied Neuropsychology, 10*(3), 153–162.

King N. S., Crawford S., Wenden, F. J., Moss, N. E., & Wade, D. T. (1995). The Rivermead post concussion symptoms questionnaire. *Journal of Neurology, 242*(9), 587–592.

Langlois J. A., Rutland-Brown, W., & Thomas, K. E. (2006). *Traumatic brain injury in the United States: Emergency department visits, hospitalizations, and deaths.* Atlanta, GA: Centers for Disease Control and Prevention.

Legome, E., & Wu, T. (2006). *Postconcussive syndrome.* Retrieved September 6, 2008, from http://www.emedicine.com/EMERG/topic865.htm

Northeast Center for Special Care. (2007). *Rancho Los Amigos Cognitive Scale* (n.d.). Retrieved May 27, 2009, from http://www.northeastcenter.com/rancho_los_amigos.htm

Pangilinan, P. H. (2008). *Classification and complications of traumatic brain injury.* Retrieved September 6, 2008, from http://www.emedicine.com/pmr/topic213.htm

Parcell, D. L., Ponsford, J. L., & Rajaratnam, S. M., Redman, J. R. (2006). Self-reported changes to nighttime sleep after traumatic brain injury. *Archives of Physical Medicine and Rehabilitation, 87*(2), 278–285.

Rappaport, M., Hall, K. M., Hopkins, H. K., Belleza, T., & Cope, D. N.. (1982). Disability rating scale for severe head trauma: Coma to community. *Archives of Physical Medicine and Rehabilitation, 63*, 118–123.

Springhouse. (2007). *Alarming signs and symptoms: Lippincott manual of nursing practice.* Philadelphia: Lippincott Williams & Wilkins.

Szaflarski, J. (2006, April 6). Study supports theory why brain-injured children often recover. *Science Daily.* Retrieved September 7, 2008, from http://www.sciencedaily.com/releases/2006/04/060406102527.htm

Teasdale, G., & Jennett, B. (1974). Assessment of coma and impaired consciousness. A practical scale. *Lancet, 13*(2), 81–84.

Turkstra, L. S., & Burgess, S. (2007). Social skills intervention for adolescents with TBI. *Perspectives on Neurophysiology and Neurogenic Speech and Language Disorders, 17*(3), 15–20.

Wade, S. L., Wolfe, C. R., Brown, T. M., & Pestian, J. P. (2005). Can a web-based family problem-solving intervention work for children with traumatic brain injury? *Rehabilitation Psychology, 50*(4), 337–345.

Webb, W. G. & Adler, R. K. (2008). *Neurology for the speech-language pathologist* (5th ed.). St. Louis, MO: Mosby Elsevier.

Wiseman-Hakes, C., Stewart, M. L., Wasserman, R., & Schuller, R. (1998). Peer group training in pragmatic skills in adolescents with acquired brain injury. *Journal of Head Trauma Rehabilitation, 13*(6), 23–38.

Ylvisaker, M., Szekeres, S. F., & Feeney, T. (2008). Communication disorders associated with traumatic brain injury. In R. Chapey (Ed.), *Language intervention strategies in aphasia and related neurogenic communication disorders* (5th ed., pp. 917–918). Philadelphia: Lippincott Williams & Wilkins.

Ylvisaker, M., Turkstra, L. S., Coelho, C., Kennedy, M. R. T., Yorkston, K., Sohlber, M. M., et al. (2007). Behavioral interventions for children and adults with behavior disorders after TBI: A systematic review of the evidence. *Brain Injury, 21*(8), 769–805.

Chapter 8
DEMENTIA

Characteristics

Dementia is classified as a syndrome in that it is characterized by a constellation of symptoms (Bayles & Tomoeda, 2007). Individuals who are diagnosed with dementia have multiple cognitive deficits. Dementia can result from various etiologies such as cerebrovascular disease, Alzheimer's disease, HIV disease, Parkinson's disease, Huntington's disease, Pick's disease, Creutzfeldt-Jakob disease, head trauma, or other medical conditions including substance-induced dementia. Individuals with a diagnosis of dementia must exhibit memory impairment and may exhibit one or more of the following symptoms: aphasia, agnosia, apraxia, and/or impaired executive functions, significant enough to affect occupational and social functioning (American Psychiatric Association, 2004). The incidences of dementia are increasing. Part of this is due to the fact that people are living longer and it is estimated that by the year 2050, 14 million Americans will be diagnosed with Alzheimer's dementia. As recently as 30 years ago, dementia was unfamiliar to most Americans, including speech-language pathologists (Bayles & Tomoeda, 2007).

The incidence of dementia is relatively high in the population. One out of 10 people over the age of 65 suffers from some form of dementia and almost 50% of those over 85 demonstrate this type of intellectual deficit. According to the DSM-IV-TR (Diagnostic and Statistical Manual of Mental Disorders-Text Revision), the individual must have a memory impairment and at least one of the following cognitive deficits for a diagnosis of dementia (American Psychiatric Association, 2004). These include:

a. aphasia—deterioration of language functions including naming
b. apraxia—difficulty executing motor activities although motor skills, sensory functions, and comprehension are intact
c. agnosia—failure to recognize or identify objects despite intact sensory function
d. disturbance in executive functioning—difficulty thinking abstractly, and planning, initiation, sequencing, and monitoring deficits

Diagnostic Factors

Dementia is usually diagnosed long after its initial onset. The first symptoms are generally memory difficulties and forgetfulness. One diagnostic challenge is to differentiate mild dementia from cognitive decline due to depression (pseudo dementia). Radiologic imaging such as CAT scan, lab tests, and neuropsychological assessment may help differentiate and identify dementia versus other disease processes than can mimic dementia. A more recently developed diagnostic screening test is now available, called the Electrical Alzheimer's Test (Warner, 2003). Electrodes for an electroencephalogram are placed on the head and spine of the patient to detect changes in the brain's electrical functions. It takes about 15 minutes to administer and can be done as an outpatient. The electroencephalogram (EEG) measures a person's P300 latency (event-related evoked potentials) to determine if it is normal. The P300 latency reflects information processing of cognitive events.

As Alzheimer's disease begins as a slowing of the brain's processing speed, this test has been found useful in detecting signs of cognitive decline before they are manifested clinically. There is some speculation that this is generated in the frontal, temporal, and parietal lobes. In people with early stage dementia, P300 latency is in excess of 400 msec, although a prolonged P300 latency does occur with normal aging. According to Barclay (2003), P300 may be one test subtle enough to identify changes in the brain before documentation of memory loss. Whereas age, memory, and mental status impairment have been well established, it is not consistently accepted that the neurodevelopment patterns of the P300 component are an electrophysiologic memory marker.

Neuropsychologists, speech-language pathologists, and other clinicians must evaluate individuals with suspected dementia. A case history including an interview with a significant others, is advised because they are most familiar with the patient and can report any memory problems or word finding difficulties that they observe. Premorbid intelligence is another important factor to consider so that the clinician can compare the patient's current functioning to his or her pre-morbid status. Hearing loss, impaired vision, depression, and medication usage are just a few additional pieces of information that must be taken into consideration when assessing a person's mental status (Hopper & Bayles, 2008). According to Hopper and Bayles (2008), a comprehensive battery of tests to assess communicative functions must be administered. Cognitive abilities including memory must be assessed. Below is a summary of selected assessment measures for dementia:

- Arizona Battery for Communication Disorders of Dementia (ABCD), Story Retelling Subtest for screening purposes (Bayles & Tomoeda, 1993)
- FAS Verbal Fluency Test (Borkowski, Benton, & Spreen, 1967)
- Mini-Mental State Examination (Folstein, Folstein, & McHugh, 1975) to screen attention, concentration, language, and memory
- Global Deterioration Scale (Reisberg, Ferris, de Leon, & Crook, 1982)

- Boston Naming Test (Kaplan, Goodglass & Weintraub, 1983)
- Boston Diagnostic Aphasia Examination-3 (Goodglass, Kaplan, & Barresi, 2000)
- The Functional Linguistic Communication Inventory (Bayles & Tomoeda, 1994)
- Western Aphasia Battery-Revised (Kertesz, 2006)
- Clinical Dementia Rating Scale (Hughes, Berg, Danziger, Coben, & Martin, 1982)
- Global Deterioration Scale (Reisberg, Ferris, de Leon, & Crook, 1982)

Dementia has both irreversible and reversible etiologies. The most familiar causes of irreversible dementia include Alzheimer's disease, Huntington's disease, vascular disease, and Parkinson's disease, fronto-temporal-parietal dementia, Creutzfeldt-Jakob disease, and Lewy body disease. For a more extensive review of the dementias see Bayles and Tomoeda, 2007. Fifty percent of those with dementia have Alzheimer's type and 20% have vascular dementia due to multiple infracts and vascular disease. The average life expectancy for a patient with Alzheimer's disease is typically eight years although it can also go on for 12 years or more. However, rapid decline is linked to three characteristics: early onset, delusions or hallucinations, or extrapyramidal signs. In these patients, small, lacunar infarcts are chronic, closing down the microvessels in the cortical and subcortical arterial system, thereby compromising function in the areas of respective distribution. The causes of reversible dementia include, but are not limited to, drug toxicity, vitamin deficiency, infections and tumors, normal pressure hydrocephalus, renal failure, congestive heart failure, and thyroid disease.

Stages of Dementia

There are typically three stages in dementia classification: early, middle, and late. Abilities change in the areas of cognition and memory, self-care, communication, and physical and sensory abilities as dementia progresses. In most instances, the individual's decline is gradual and insidious, occurring over a six-year period of time before there is any clinical evidence (Collie & Maruff, 2000).

Early Stage Dementia

In early stages of dementia (generally referring to Alzheimer's dementia), the person's ability to communicate depends on their recent memory. Consequently, they can define words and describe pictures but may have difficulty following a line of conversation. However, they still may have the ability to but follow a 3-step command (Figure 8–1). Some of their sentences remain incomplete and they may repeat themselves. Comprehension of longer material may be reduced. Reading and writing at this stage are often spared but spelling errors are common. Syntax is normal. Decreases in psychomotor speed, perceptual speed, abstract reasoning, visuospatial performance, and episodic memory are typically seen in early stages (Bayles, 2004). From a functional standpoint the person with early stage dementia often has minimal difficulty with activities of daily living; however, one may observe a decline in the following areas:

■ Difficulty handling finances
■ Disoriented to time and place
■ Episodic and working memory difficulties including recalling personal information
■ Difficulty with complex tasks
■ Decreased awareness of recent events

■ Disjointed conversation (cohesion and content)
■ Mild semantic dysnomia (apple for pear, pen for pencil, etc.)
■ Mini-Mental State Exam (score 16–24 of 30)

Middle Stage Dementia

In the middle stage of dementia, people may be disoriented to time and place. The individual can usually name items when given confrontation naming tasks but has difficulty engaging in conversation. Verbal output tends to have less meaning. Syntax remains intact but sentence fragments are common. Comprehension for two-step commands is generally accomplished but three steps tend to be difficult. Writing words to dictation is often intact however writing any lengthy material is difficult (Bayles, 2004). The individual may still be able to read but they often forget what they read. The following symptoms may be present:

■ Disoriented for time and place
■ Restlessness and distractibility are common
■ Poor episodic memory with lack of awareness for recent events
■ Encoding and retrieval deficits

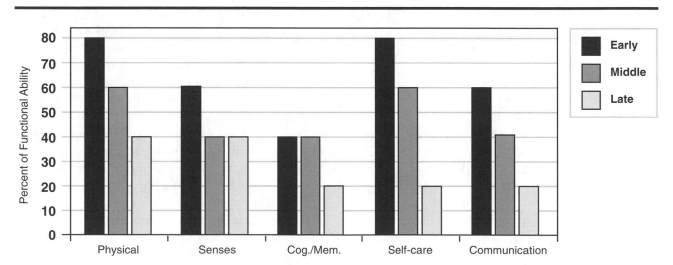

Figure 8–1. Abilities and stages of dementia. From The Source® for Alzheimer's and Dementia by Pam Reese © 2000, Reprinted with permission of LinguiSystems, Inc.

- Poor semantic memory
- Poor attention and focus
- Visual perception and constructional deficits
- Cognitive deficits
- Forgetfulness for common information
- Greater knowledge about remote past than present
- Assistance is needed with ADLs (activities of daily living)
- Verbal output is fluent but slower and less informative with word-finding problems
- Agitation and anxiety may be present
- Reading and writing are impaired
- Mini-Mental State Exam Scores (8–15 of 30)

Late Stage Dementia

In the late stage of dementia there is extensive memory loss. The individual is disoriented for time, place, and factors relating to self. Problem-solving abilities are very limited. Minimal functional vocabulary may remain. Most remaining language consists of either common social phrases or nonsense. Some people become mute. However, many can still follow a simple one-step command and read a basic word (Bayles, 2004). At this point, they often become incontinent and they have difficulty walking. The following characteristics are typically seen at this late stage:

- Disoriented for person, place, and time
- Very severe cognitive deficits
- In very late stage, person may be non-ambulatory
- Severe impairment in working and declarative memory
- Verbal output is diminished and communication is out of context but grammar is generally intact
- All verbal abilities may be lost (esp. in patients who are bladder and bowel incontinent) and person may be mute
- For those who are only bladder incontinent, they may be able to respond to greetings, recognize their written name, recognize common drawn objects, and follow single-step directions (Bayles, Tomoeda, Cruz, & Mahendra, 2000)

- Common language deficits are reflected in being mute, perseverative, echolalic, and palilalic (excessive repetitive utterances)
- Scores on Mini-Mental State Exam (0–9 of 30)

Memory Systems and Dementia

In order to understand the nature of dementia and its effects on the lives of patients and their families, it is helpful to become familiar with the memory systems at work in normal and impaired cognition. Memory has been defined as representations that are stored through a process of encoding, consolidation and retrieval for acquisition and manipulation of knowledge (Baddeley, 1999). The discussion below describes the relationships among the three primary areas of memory: sensory memory, working memory, and long-term memory.

Sensations come into the peripheral nervous system and may enter consciousness. Sensory memory lasts from less than one second to a maximum of two seconds. If sensory information enters conscious awareness, sensation is attended to and can then be interpreted. Previous experiences assist in the interpretation and meaning of the stimuli.

Multiple systems are involved in memory. Short-term memory, also referred to as working memory, requires attention and concentration to remember or retain information.

Baddeley (2002) reviewed his model of a limited capacity system for temporary storage of information and expanded it to include the episodic buffer. In his system, the visuospatial sketchpad holds visual images while the phonological loop temporarily stores verbal information. The central executive manages these subsystems by apportioning attention to them. Therefore, a person can hold a concept, word, picture, or idea in memory and manipulate it to solve problems (Baddeley, 1983; Fockert, Rees, Frith, & Lavie, 2001). The system serves as a link between working memory and long-term memory so that new information can be stored as an episode and later retrieved (Baddeley, 2002).

Long-term memory involves declarative knowledge of factual information (also known as declarative or explicit memory) and nondeclarative memory (also known as implicit memory) which refers to motor memories and conditioned responses (Squire, 1995). Working memory processes information from long-term memory. Diseases that affect cortical areas generally affect declarative memory. Diseases that affect subcortical structures (i.e., basal ganglia) generally produce nondeclarative memory deficits (Hopper & Bayles, 2008). Table 8–1 presents a breakdown of memory deficits.

Types of Dementia

Vascular Dementia (VaD)

Vascular dementia is the second most common cause of dementia. People with hypertension, atherosclerosis, and a history of previous strokes are all at risk for this acquiring this type of dementia. Vascular dementia is usually caused by ischemia or a restriction of blood flow in the vessels of the brain. Those patients who demonstrate symptoms consis-

tent with dementia after sustaining multiple deep, lacunar strokes, are usually diagnosed with multi-infarct dementia. It is possible to develop a vascular dementia secondary to large cerebral infracts, ischemic events, and/or microvascular disease, i.e., the occlusion of the fine capillaries within the cortex. Approximately one-fourth to one-third of patients who have had one or more ischemic stroke develops vascular dementia within 3 months (Pohjasvaara, Erkinjuntti, et.al., 1998).

Dementia of the Alzheimer's Type (DAT)

More commonly known as Alzheimer's disease, this is by far the most common type of dementia observed in the population. It was also known as presenile dementia, as its onset can be seen in the fifth decade, unlike senile dementia which is associated with normal aging. The cognitive-linguistic, affective, and behavioral aspects of each type are similar, however. On autopsy, the brain of the person with DAT will

Table 8–1. Declarative and Nondeclarative Memory Systems

Declarative Memory (Explicit)	Nondeclarative Memory (Implicit)
Semantic (Concepts) • Involves conceptual knowledge and understanding of constructs from which people organize their world and experiences.	Procedural (Motor Skills) • Involves learned skills that become automatic with practice and repetition (riding a bike).
Episodic (Events) • This ability is "most affected early on in dementia." This autobiographic system receives and stores information about events that people experience.	Procedural (Verbal & Cognitive Skills) • Involves learned skills that occur without conscious awareness such as knowing how to get information to someone through the mail.
Lexical (Words) • Memory for words, their meanings, spelling, and pronunciation. These are the linguistic representations of concepts.	Priming • Associations are made so that earlier experiences trigger words, thoughts, and memories of similar experience.
	Conditioned Responses • A reaction to a previous similar stimulus occurs due to a chain of associated triggers. Habits are often developed because of associations for events that are repeated.

show changes in the association areas of the parietal, temporal, and frontal lobes, as well as in the hippocampus, a major structure for memory. DAT tends to begin in the hippocampal area which is essential to forming episodic memories. This is why individuals in early stages have difficulty recalling recent events. As the disease progresses to the frontal region and temporoparietal regions of the brain, declarative memory is affected for semantic and lexical memories and the person will have difficulty organizing information and recalling words and concepts. The basal ganglia and motor cortex are not impacted throughout most of the disease's progression and, therefore, procedural memory often remains intact (Bayles, 2004). Autopsied brains also reveal neuronal plaques, neurofibrillary tangles, and granulovascular degeneration, which are all abnormal tissue changes. Although tangles and plaques lead to cell death and impact intercellular transmission, subcortical structures and the motor strip remain unaffected. Therefore, the speech of individuals with DAT generally is spared (Bayles, 2004). The brain's biochemistry also degenerates in these patients, in that there is a reduction in the function of the cholinergic and noradrenergic systems that disrupt nerve transmission. Unfortunately, the etiology of DAT is not certain. Some educated guesses include aluminum toxicity, immune dysfunction, and viral infection with a possible genetic component.

Parkinson's Dementia

The dementia associated with Parkinson's disease (PD) is not observed until the very late stages of the disease process. Parkinson's disease is a neurodegenerative disease with complex motor disturbances due to a loss of striatal dopaminergic neurons in the substantia nigra. Typical features of the motoric aspect of this disease are slow movements (bradykinesia), rigidity, pin wheeling, tremor, a masked-like face, and disturbances in gait (festinating), posture, and balance. Treatments for PD include dopamine to restore that neurotransmitter to optimal levels and deep brain stimulation (DBT). According to Bayles (2004), individuals with PD have motor speech difficulties due to damage of

the basal ganglia and striatal-cortical circuits as well as deficits in memory, attention, and executive functioning. However, knowledge for language, including sentence comprehension and confrontation naming, tends to be preserved.

Individuals at the end stage of PD can manifest with cognitive changes consistent with dementia although the best estimate indicates that approximately 29% of all patients develop it (Marttila & Rinne, 1976). The etiology of the dementia in PD is still debated. Some researchers believe that it is due to cortical degeneration and others to subcortical degeneration that impairs the neurologic control of attention (Brown & Marsden, 1988). Rinne, Portin, et al. (2000) reported that there was reduced fluorodopa uptake in PD individuals in the caudate nucleus and the frontal cortex. They stated that this impairs performance on any tests that require executive functions. Regardless of etiology, PD patients who do develop dementia have problems communicating due to deficits in memory, attention, and the higher level executive functions (Bayles, 2004).

Frontal-Temporal-Parietal Dementias (FTP)

Frontal lobe dementias are rare (fewer than 10% of all diagnosed cases of dementia). This type of dementia typically has a very early onset, usually in the fourth or fifth decade of a person's life. It is primarily associated with personality changes, reduced language abilities, and difficulty executing complex tasks. People with this type of dementia will become moody, self-centered, and unable to be empathic. They may appear unfeeling. A true diagnosis can only be made upon autopsy. Under those conditions, the brain will reveal significant cell loss in the frontal and temporal cortices.

Pick's disease is a type of frontal lobe dementia, with characteristics that set it apart from the more general type described above. Neary et al. (1988) suggest that Pick's disease is a variant form of FTP dementia (Neary, Snoden, et. al., 1988). It is also rare, seen predominantly in women, with an incidence 1/10th as much as that of DAT. The etiology of Pick's dementia is due to the loss of neurons, gliosis, and neuronal inclusions called Pick bodies. The pattern of degeneration in these patients is different from that of FTP or DAT. In the case of the Pick's patient, the neuronal deterioration is primarily frontal but includes the inferior motor area and the anterior temporal lobes. Pick's disease and DAT both share one similar structural feature: the deterioration of the hippocampus and the amygdaloid nucleus.

The FTP dementias, including Pick's, have characteristic cognitive, behavioral, and language features. Behaviorally, these patients will demonstrate reduced spontaneity, reduced insight, and reduced executive functions. Their language abnormalities will be noted early in the process, unlike DAT. These patients will have reduced initiation, palilalia, echolalia, and logorrhea (more so in Pick's). Mutism can also be observed in middle to late stage Pick's disease.

Creutzfeldt-Jakob Disease

Creutzfeldt-Jakob disease is caused by the presence of prions. Prions are unconventional, transmissible agents (not a virus or a bacterium). They are a special type of protein that can be transmitted from one animal to another. They can cause a group of degenerative diseases of the nervous system. These diseases can be manifest as sporadic, infectious, or inherited disorders. Only about 15% of cases have a genetic link. Creutzfeldt-Jakob disease (CJD) is defined by the American Medical Association as:

A rare transmissible encephalopathy most prevalent between the ages of 50 and 70 years. Affected individuals may present with sleep disturbances, personality changes, ataxia, aphasia, visual loss, weakness, muscle atrophy, myoclonus, progressive dementia, and death within one year of disease onset.

A familial form exhibiting autosomal dominant inheritance and a new variant (potentially associated with encephalopathy, bovine spongiform) have been described. Pathologic features include prominent cerebellar and cerebral cortical spongiform degeneration and the presence of prions (Johnson & Gibbs, 1998). The prognosis for these patients is not favorable. They usually expire within one year of the diagnosis. As noted in the AMA definition above, these patients will have symptoms consistent with aphasia.

Huntington's Disease

Huntington's disease (HD), also known as Huntington's chorea, is a progressive and fatal neurodegenerative disease. It is a genetic disease (autosomal dominant), characterized by choreoathetoid movements and dementia. The incidence of HD in the population is approximately 5 per 100,000 and affects people of northern European descent. The age of onset is in one's thirties or forties. The initial symptoms are personality changes and sometimes frank psychosis, with depression being a very common feature. This neurodegenerative disease is classified as a hyperkinetic movement disorder, hence the choreoathetoid movements.

Communication and cognitive functions are both affected by HD. Early after onset, the patient begins to manifest characteristics of a hyperkinetic dysarthria and HD patients are often nonverbal during the end stage of the disease process. Language deficits associated with HD include difficulty initiating conversational speech, formulation problems, word finding problems, poor auditory processing for complex material, and slow response time. They also can demonstrate reading and writing problems. Cognitively, they have difficulty learning new information and new tasks, exhibit reduced executive functions, and poor attention and concentration (Klasner, n.d.).

All of these difficulties can be and usually are present in one individual. They often begin in a mild form and become more severe as the disease progresses. Abilities are often unpredictable, because deficits occur randomly during the general progression of the disease. This unpredictability creates more coping difficulties for the Huntington's disease patient, because he/she cannot rely on having or maintaining various skills at any given time. For example, the Huntington's disease patient could make a request clearly at one moment, but then have tremendous difficulty articulating that same request a moment later.

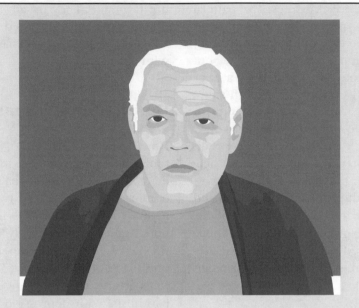

Case Scenario: Max

History and Physical (H & P): A 76-year-old Caucasian male who presented to a neurologist on consult from his primary physician as an outpatient. The patient was brought in by his wife who reported problems with simple calculations, telling time, and home repair tasks, that were normally simple and routine for him to do.

Past Medical History (PMH): Cardiomyopathy; cortical atrophy noted on last MRI with enlarged sulci; hypercholesterolemia; family reported difficulty with numbers and time for approximately 6 months PTA (prior to this admission).

Social History: Self-employed in a trucking business; married with two grown children in the area. Some postsecondary education (Associate's Degree); naval officer during WWII. Family reported that patient is "less moody" over the past few months.

Surgical History: Hernia repair.

A Functional Analysis of Max's Dementia

Max's ability to understand and use language is intact for his ADL needs. However, he has difficulty formulating language to discuss recent events and facts, dates and time, facts of general knowledge related to his personal history, and political and social history of the times. His semantic memory is also beginning to show signs of decline, manifested by semantic paraphasias. There are concomitant word-finding problems. Max's procedural memory is still intact, so he can perform basic meal preparation, gardening, and minor home repairs. However, due to his attentional deficits, his safety at home and in public can be compromised. This can lead to dangerous errors while executing activities of daily living.

Language Expression	**Automatic Speech:** WFL	**Repetition Ability:** WFL	**Lexical Retrieval-Naming:** Naming difficulties noted; specifically names of people and locations; poor confrontation naming.	**Conversational Ability:** Common social phrases were used appropriately; able to express his wants and needs at the sentence level; able to engage in a one-on-one dialogue that was concrete, and context driven (contextualized language); narrative discourse focused on two topics: lack of income and returning to work; patient could be re-directed with verbal cue.	**Pragmatic Skills:** WFL — **Paraphasias:** Semantic paraphasias noted in conversation.
Speech	**Rate:** WFL	**Intelligibility:** WFL	**Prosody:** WFL	**Articulation:** WFL	**Fluency:** WFL
Auditory Comprehension	**Answering Yes/No Questions:** Answers to abstract yes/no questions were mildly impaired.	**Executing Commands:** WFL executing one-step commands was WFL; following complex multi-step questions was mild-moderately impaired.	**Understanding Stories & Paragraphs:** WFL for short paragraphs up to 5 sentences in length. Errors increase as paragraph increases.	**Understanding Conversational Speech:** Sentence comprehension was WFL; comprehension at the conversational level was variable depending on the number of people involved and the complexity of the information.	**Identifying Objects & their Functions:** WFL
Reading	**Word-level Comprehension:** WFL	**Sentence-level Comprehension:** Good for simple declarative sentences; moderately impaired as the semantic and syntactic complexity increased, e.g., connectives and clausal relationships.	**Oral Reading:** WFL for simple, commonly used high frequency words and simple declarative sentences.	**Oral Spelling:** Moderately impaired for irregularly spelled words and polysyllabic words.	
Written Expression	**Copying:** Able to copy words and sentences.	**Writing to Dictation:** Able to write sentences to dictation.	**Self-generated:** Writes functionally at the phrase level to express his needs if necessary.	**Written Spelling:** Moderately impaired for irregularly spelled words and polysyllabic words characterized by missing letters.	**Drawing:** Not functional for communication purposes and often ended up in preservative "doodles".
Cognition	**Alertness:** Level of alertness during daytime hours was WFL; Sometimes awakens fully alert and agitated in the middle of the night asking to go to his adult day-care program.	**Attention/Concentration:** Mild-moderately impaired raising the issue of safety at home and in public.	**Visuospatial Skills:** Patient was unable to consistently recognize family members and thought they were impostors.	**Memory:** Semantic memory is moderately impaired; moderately- severely impaired episodic memory for recent events; procedural memory is functional for over-learned tasks, e.g., gardening, minor home repairs, meal preparation.	**Executive Functions:** Relied on family members to make appointments; unable to plan and organize a daily task independently; poor judgment for home safety scenarios.
Behavioral Symptoms	**Deficit awareness:** "There is something wrong with my brain. It's like there's a hole in it".	**Frustration:** Agitation and anxiety noted; more agitated at night.	**Emotional Lability:** Not noted.	**Current Personality Characteristics:** Pre-morbidly rigid, confident, assertive and rule-bound (ex-military officer); currently, more dependent, frightened, still inflexible.	

Figure 8–2. Diagnostic profile for Max.

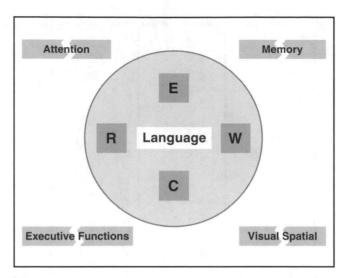

Figure 8–3. ALD Target Model for Max.

Max is able to write sentences to dictation, but can only use writing functionally at the phrase level to express his needs if necessary. His reading comprehension is good for sentences, but is moderately impaired at the more complex paragraph level. This will preclude Max from reading and understanding any detailed written instructions. Training the family to give Max written instructions at the short phrase level, supplemented by pictures and/or symbols, is suggested. For example, a written note placed above the sink, "Rinse off dishes" paired with a picture or drawing of a dish being washed, may facilitate clean-up. Due to the fact that this is a progressive and degenerative disease, the family is advised to manipulate the environment for Max's comfort and ease. Communication with Max is best when it is about the here and now, supplemented by tangible objects relevant to the context. Max's wife, the primary caretaker, is encouraged to reduce her rate of speech and allow time for him to process and respond. It is also recommended that she not call attention to his difficulties because he does not have the ability to repair his errors. She must also be instructed to reduce the number of people participating in a conversation when Max is present. In general, indirect therapy is most appropriate for Max at this stage of his dementia with a focus on counseling and education of his family regarding the goals and procedures of this therapeutic approach. The clinician can also consider the FOCUSED Caregiver Training Program by Ripich, Ziol, et al. (1999) if more formal intervention is desired. Finally, Max's wife may benefit from a support group for families dealing with dementia.

Critical Thinking/Learning Activity

■ What information indicates that this is a person with dementia?
■ How would this patient's prosopagnosia impact communicative effectiveness with his family members?

■ What are the family counseling and education issues in this case, and how would you address them?

■ What can you do to facilitate auditory processing when Max is part of a group of people having a conversation?

■ Write a SOAP note on this patient. Assume that you are seeing him for the first time after the evaluation session. Include three short-term therapeutic objectives in your note.

Treatment Considerations

Max was diagnosed with dementia of the Alzheimer's type. He tries to participate in conversations but demonstrates frustration when he is unable to do so effectively. Consequently, he withdraws into silence. His language is comprised primarily of idioms, common social phrases, and stereotypic utterances. Due to his memory impairments and inability to drive safely, Max is very dependent on his wife for transportation to appointments. He often wakes his wife during the night thinking that it is, "time to leave." Max has some awareness of his deficits, and told his daughter, "There's something wrong in my head." When out in the community he often develops uncharacteristic impatience and has difficulty staying in one place for more than 15 minutes. Max is most affected by his cognitive rather than linguistic problems. He can still communicate with his family and friends effectively enough to have his daily wants and needs met. Consequently, Max's therapy must focus primarily on his cognitive deficits and secondarily on his minor linguistic impairments. However, the clinician must keep in mind that dementia is a progressive disease process so Max's therapy must change as he does, with different accommodations set according to his needs. There are various treatment programs and therapeutic techniques specific to dementia that the clinician can employ, which we describe next.

Some Therapeutic Options

We suggest that the speech-language pathologist consider the following selected programs when planning therapy for people with dementia:

■ Spaced-Retrieval Training (SRT) (Camp & Schaller, 1989; Hopper et al., 2005). SRT uses a verbally mediated technique to help with safety and activities of daily living. The patient rehearses a specific response or action to a stimulus across repeated trials. The time between the presentation of the stimulus and the request from the clinician for the response is gradually increased. The patient eventually learns the new behavior. For example, putting on a pair of pants requires certain steps to accomplish the act. The SLP would use Spaced Retrieval Training to facilitate the learning of these steps (Camp, Foss, O'Hanlon, & Stevens, 1996).

- FOCUSED Caregiver Training Program (Ripich, Ziol, et al., 1999). Family/caregiver counseling and education is a cornerstone of treatment with people with dementia. The clinician must educate the family/caregivers about the disease process itself, the goals and procedures of therapy, and their role in the treatment plan. The SLP also must counsel them around the issues of living with a person with dementia and the impact it can have on their daily life due to the cognitive-linguistic deficits inherent to dementia as wells as its progressive nature. One program specific to family and/or caregiver training, supporting functional communication is FOCUSED (Ripich, 1994). In this approach, the suggestions for communication enrichment follow the acronym. The F is for *Face-to-Face* communication; O reminds the communication partner to *Orient* the patient to the topic; C refers to keeping the continuity of the topic *Concrete*; U helps remind the conversational partner to help *Unstick* any communication blocks; S refers to *Structure* in using yes/no and direct choice question; E is to support and encourage an *Exchange* in conversation; and D refers to the importance of using *Direct*, short, and simple sentences when speaking to the person with dementia.
- Stimulus generalization (Thompson, 1989). The clinician can use a *Stimulus generalization* approach to treat persons with dementia. In this approach, a trained response from the treatment session is generalized to a new context where there may be different people, materials, or places. For example, the person with dementia may learn to ask for clarification when he or she does not understand what is said during the therapy session. The therapy teaches the patient to transfer this new behavior to a new context, that is, at home, the physician's office (Thompson, 1989).
- External memory aids (Reese, 2000). *Memory books and daily logs* can be used to optimize the patient's ability to perform his or her activities of daily living. The clinician facilitates the patient's completion of the daily log and discusses the content. The use of photographs from the patient's life may also enhance quality of life and augment communication due to the familiarity of the contextual references. Any of these activities can be used to address semantic and word retrieval goals. Therapeutic approaches address cognitive-communicative impairment (Helm-Estabrooks, 1995).
- Strength-based communication and programming. (Eisner, 2001).
- Validation Therapy (Feil, 1991). Validate through words and gestures to review what the person says, regardless of fact (Toseland, Diehl, et.al., 1997).
- Graphic & Written Cues (Hoerster, Hickey, & Bourgeois, 2001). Provide written information and photos to support recognition memory; use a memory wallet, book, or daily log.
- Montessori-based Interventions (Orsulic-Jeras, Schneider, & Camp, 2000).
- Create structured and stimulating activities for engagement and social interaction.

References

American Psychiatric Association. (2004). *Diagnostic and statistical manual of mental disorders (DSM-IV-TR)* (4th ed., text revision). Washington, DC: Author.

Baddeley, A. D. (1983). Working memory. *Philosophical Transactions of the Royal Society of London. Series B, Biological Sciences, 302*(1110), 311-324.

Baddeley, A. D. (1999). *Essentials of human memory.* Hove, East Sussex: Psychology Press.

Baddeley, A. D. (2002). Is working memory still working? *European Psychologist, 7*(2), 85-97.

Barclay, L. (2003). P300 latency accurately predicts memory impairment. *Clinical Electroencephalography, 34*, 124-139.

Bayles, K. (2004). Dementia. In R. Kent (Ed.), *The MIT encyclopedia of communication disorders.* Cambridge, MA: A Bradford Book.

Bayles, K., & Tomoeda, C. (1993). *Arizona battery for communication disorders of dementia.* Austin, TX: Pro-Ed.

Bayles, K., & Tomoeda, C. (2007). *Cognitive-communication disorders of dementia.* San Diego, CA: Plural.

Bayles, K., Tomoeda, C., Cruz, R., & Mahendra, N. (2000). Communication abilities of individuals with late-stage Alzheimer disease. *Alzheimer Disease and Associated Disorders, 14*(3), 176-181.

Bayles, K. A., & Tomoeda, C. K. (1994). *The functional linguistic communication inventory.* Austin, TX: Pro-Ed.

Borkowski, J. G., Benton, A. L., & Spreen, O. (1967). Word fluency and brain damage. *Neuropsychologia, 5*, 135-140.

Brown, R. G., & Marsden, C. D. (1988). Internal and external cues and the control of attention in Parkinson's disease. *Brain, 111*, 323-345.

Camp, C., & Schaller, J. (1989). Epilogue: Spaced-retrieval memory training in an adult day-care center. *Educational Gerontology, 15*(6), 641-648.

Camp, C. J., Foss, J. W., O'Hanlon, A. M., & Stevens, A. B. (1996). Memory intervention for persons with dementia. *Applied Cognitive Psychology, 10*, 193-210.

Collie, A., & Maruff, P. (2000). The neuropsychology of pre-clinical Alzheimer's disease and mild cognitive impairment. *Neuroscience and Biobehavioral Reviews, 24*(3), 365-374.

Eisner, E. (2001). *Can do activities for adults with Alzheimer's disease.* Austin, TX: Pro-Ed.

Feil, N. (1991). Validation therapy. In P. K. H. Kim (Ed.), *Serving the elderly: Skills for practice* (pp. 89-116). Edison, NJ: Aldine Transaction.

Folstein, M. F., Folstein, S. E., & McHugh, P. R. (1975). "Mini-mental state." A practical method for grading the cognitive state of patients for the clinician. *Journal of Psychiatric Research, 12*(3), 189-198.

Fockert, J. W., Rees, G., Frith, C. D., & Lavie, N. (2001). The role of working memory in visual selective attention. *Science, 291*, 1803-1806.

Goodglass, H., Kaplan, E., & Barresi, B. (2000). *Boston Diagnostic Aphasia Examination* (3rd Ed.). Philadelphia: Lippincott Williams & Wilkins.

Helm-Estabrooks, N. (1995). *Cognitive-linguistic task book.* Sandwich, MA: Cape Cod Institute.

Hoerster, L., Hickey, E., Bourgeois, M. (2001). Effects of memory aids on conversations between nursing home residents with dementia and nursing assistants. *Neuropsychological Rehabilitation, 11*(3-4), 399-427.

Hopper, T., & Bayles, K. A. (2008). Management of neurogenic communication disorders associated with dementia. In R. Chapey (Ed.), *Language intervention strategies in aphasia and related neurogenic communication disorders* (5th ed.). Philadelphia: Wolters Kluwer/Lippincott Williams & Wilkins.

Hopper, T., Mahendra, N., Kim, E., Azuma, T., Bayles, K. A., Cleary, S. J., et al. (2005). Evidence-based practice recommendations for working with individuals with dementia: Spaced retrieval training. *Journal of Medical Speech-Language Pathology, 13*, 27-34.

Hughes, C., Berg, L., Danzinger, W., Coben, L., & Martin, R. (1982). *Clinical Dementia Rating Scale.* Hagerstown, MD: Lippincott Williams & Wilkins.

Johnson, R. T., & Gibbs, C. J. (1998). Creutzfeldt-Jakob disease and related transmissible spongiform encephalopathies. *New England Journal of Medicine, 339*(27), 1994-2004.

Kaplan, E., Goodglass, H., & Weintraub, S. (1983) *Boston Naming Test.* Philadelphia: Lippincott Williams & Wilkins.

Kertesz, A. (2006). *Western Aphasia Battery-Revised.* Austin, TX: Pro-Ed.

Klasner, E. (n.d.) *Huntington's disease, Fact Sheet 9, Communication Skills.* Retrieved August 22, 2008, from http://members.aol.com/hdanwlancs/Fsheet9.html

Marttila, R. J., & Rinne, U. K. (1976). Dementia in Parkinson's disease. *Acta Neurologica Scandanavica, 54*, 431-441.

Neary, D., Snoden, J. S., Northen, B., et al. (1988). Dementia of frontal lobe type. *Journal of Neurosurgery and Psychology, 51*, 353-361.

Orsulic-Jeras, S., Schneider, N. M., Camp, C. J., Nicholson, P., & Helbig, M. (2001). Montessori-based dementia activities in long-term care: Training and implementation. *Activities, Adaptation, and Aging, 25,* 107–120.

Pohjasvaara, T., Erkinjuntti, T., Ylikoski, R., Hietanen, M., Varaja, R., & Kaste, M. (1998). Clinical determinants of post stroke dementia. *Stroke, 29,* 75–81.

Reese, P. B. (2000). *The source for Alzheimer's and dementia* (p. 12). East Moline, IL: LinguaSystems.

Reisberg, B., Ferris, S. H., de Leon, M. J., & Crook, T. (1982). The global deterioration scale for assessment of primary degenerative dementia. *American Journal of Psychiatry, 139,* 1136–1139.

Rinne, J. O., Portin, R., Ruottinen, H., Nurmi, E., Bergman, J., Haaparanta, M., et al. (2000). Cognitive impairment and the brain dopaminergic system in Parkinson disease. *Archives of Neurology, 57,* 470–475.

Ripich, D. N. (1994). Functional communication training with AD patients: A caregiver training program. *Alzheimer Disease and Associated Disorders, 8*(3), 95–109.

Ripich, D. N., Ziol, E., Fritsch, T., & Durand, E. J. (1999). Training Alzheimer's disease caregivers for successful communication. *Clinical Gerontologist, 21*(1), 37–56.

Squire, L. R. (1994). Priming and multiple memory systems: Perceptual mechanisms of implicit memory. In D. L. Schacter & E. Tulving (Eds.), *Memory systems.* Cambridge, MA: MIT Press.

Thompson, C. K. (1989). Generalization in the treatment of aphasia. In L. V. McReynolds & J. Spradlin (Eds.), *Generalization strategies in the treatment of communication disorders.* Lewiston, NY: BC Decker.

Toseland, R., Diehl, M., Freeman, K., Manzanares, T., Naleppa, M., & McCallion, P. (1997). The impact of validation group therapy on nursing home residents with dementia. *Journal of Applied Gerontology, 16*(1), 31–50.

Warner, J. (2003). Current research on diagnosing dementia. *Journal of Neurology, Neurosurgery and Psychiatry, 74,* 413–414.

Chapter 9

ENCEPHALOPATHY AND ACQUIRED LANGUAGE DISORDERS

Characteristics

Encephalopathy is a nonspecific term that describes a disease or disorder of the brain. The disease causes diffuse cortical damage across both hemispheres. Cerebral dysfunction associated with encephalopathy is often due to one of the following: dehydration, hypoglycemia, metabolic dysfunctions, poor nutrition, toxic processes, diabetic ketoacidosis, drug intoxication, uremia, meningitis, bacterial infection, viral infection, or anoxia (National Institute of Neurological Disorders and Stroke, 2007). This is certainly not a comprehensive accounting of all possible etiologies leading to encephalopathy, but those listed are among the most frequently encountered in a clinical setting. The presenting feature of a progressive encephalopathy (that is not once attributable to an acute event such as cardiac arrest) is a subtle change in a person's personality, behavior, cognitive functioning, level of alertness, level of attentiveness, lethargy, and distractibility. In anoxic encephalopathy where there is an acute onset due to lack of oxygen to the brain, deterioration is more immediate. According to Shulman and Romano (1999), the highest percentage of patients with encephalopathy are found in geriatric wards. Approximately 5 to 15% are on medical-surgical floors and 20 to 30% of individuals with encephalopathy are on surgical intensive care units.

In progressive encephalopathies, one will initially notice confusion, inattentiveness, and alterations in memory and cognition. Other symptoms can include myoclonus or involuntary twitching, nystagmus (rapid involuntary eye movements), tremor, seizures, and difficulty speaking and swallowing (National Institute of Neurological Disorders and Stroke, 2007). The patient may progress from chronic confusion and hypersomnolence to delirium, and possibly even coma. If the patient becomes delirious, there may be visual delusions or hallucinations.

Organ disease is the etiology of metabolic encephalopathy. If the metabolic byproducts produced by the organs are not properly processed or biologically removed, an imbalance of magnesium, calcium, phosphorous, sodium, and/or glucose levels results thereby affecting brain functioning. To determine the cause of an encephalopathy, blood and spinal fluid are examined, and electroencephalograms and imaging studies are conducted (NINDS, 2007) (Table 9–1).

Drug and Alcohol Intoxication

Drug intoxication causes an acute change of mental status and can occur whenever there is an excess of a drug in the bloodstream. This can be due to addiction, recreational drug use or even iatrogenically caused (medically induced). It is typically associated

Table 9–1. Examples of Encephalopathies

Condition	Causes
Liver damage	Hepatic encephalopathy
Kidney damage/failure	Uremic encephalopathy
Cardiorespiratory arrest	Hypoxic/Anoxic encephalopathy
Hypertension	Hypertensive encephalopathy
Hypotension	Hypoxic encephalopathy
Cushing's syndrome	Endocrine encephalopathy
Addison's disease	Endocrine encephalopathy
Thyroid disease	Endocrine encephalopathy
Thiamine deficiency	Wernicke's encephalopathy

with drugs that have an anticholinergic effect, that is, drugs that block the uptake of acetylcholine at the synapse. The drugs most commonly associated with drug intoxication are:

- Over-the-counter cold preparations
- Antihistamines
- Antidepressants
- Neuroleptics
- Anti-Parkinson's medication
- Narcotics
- High-dose steroids
- Sedatives/tranquilizers
- Amphetamines
- Cocaine
- Hallucinogens
- Alcohol

Alcoholism is a very prevalent disease and is responsible for many hospital admissions. Therefore, the speech-language pathologist must become familiar with the clinical and cognitive manifestations of alcohol-related illness. The National Survey of Drug Use and Health found that approximately 19 million Americans were dependent on or abused alcohol in 2005. Of these, 3 million were dependent on or abused an illicit drug. Fifty-six percent of the 19 million were seen in ambulatory care settings (hospitals and clinics) (Substance Abuse and Mental Health Services Administration, Office of Applied Studies, 2006).

The person admitted to the hospital with alcohol-related illness may be in a state of delirium tremens (DT). The patient experiencing DTs is subject to perceptual hallucinations, anxiety, acute mental disorder, and sweating (diaphoresis). Typically, the patient will be placed on a thiamine IV (intravenous) drip before glucose is administered. These patients are often dehydrated and electrolyte depleted, so IV fluids are also ordered by the medical staff. Furthermore, this type of patient may have low sodium (hyponatremic) but if sodium is replaced too rapidly, there can be central pontine destruction of the myelin sheath (myelinolysis), which may result in changes to cranial nerve V (trigeminal nerve), cranial nerve VI (abducens), cranial nerve VII (facial), and cranial nerve VIII (acoustic) nerve. To prevent severe withdrawal symptoms and seizures, benzodiazepines (Valium or Xanax) are usually given.

The speech-language pathologist may be consulted to assess the patient's cognitive-linguistic status once the patient is stabilized and transferred to a medical floor.

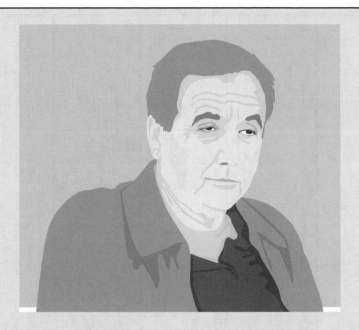

Case Scenario: Tommy

History and Physical (H & P): Tommy is a 57-year-old white male, admitted to the ED via EMS s/p being found down (breathing but unconscious at the scene) outside of a bar in his neighborhood. His blood pressure (BP) was 86/34 with a heart rate (HR) of 130; intubated prophylactically by EMS; vital signs stabilized in ED; diagnosed with alcohol poisoning.

Past Medical History (PMH): Severe alcoholism; HTN (hypertension); Hepatitis B and C; IDDM (insulin dependent diabetes mellitus); pancreatitis; multiple hospitalizations for alcohol-related illnesses and injuries; undocumented history of cocaine abuse (per wife's report patient did use the drug "about two years ago, then went back to drinking heavily").

Social History: Former truck driver but hasn't worked since the age of 50 due to revocation of his CDL (commercial driver's license). Pt. has 5 children, ages 21 to 35, all in the area. Lives with wife in first floor apartment five steps to enter. Wife works full-time in a factory. He smokes 2 to 3 packs of cigarettes per day. The patient completed 11th grade. Patient's interests include "anything about 'Nam" according to wife. Patient was a Vietnam War veteran and was active in his VFW post.

Surgical History: s/p cholecycstectomy (removal of gall bladder).

A Functional Analysis of Tommy's Encephalopathy

At the time of the assessment, Tommy's ability to understand language was intact for grammatically simple utterances at the conversational level. As sentence complexity increased, his comprehension diminished. This affected Tommy's ability to participate in the social milieu of his environment. His expressive language,

Language Expression

Automatic Speech:	Repetition Ability:	Lexical Retrieval-Naming:	Conversational Ability:	Pragmatic Skills:	Paraphasias:
WFL	WFL	WFL	Able to express his wants and needs at the sentence level; able to engage in one-on-one dialogue; narrative discourse was not focused due to tangential speech.	Poor topic maintenance; tangential output causes interrupted discourse; inappropriate pauses; turn-taking impaired; frequently interrupts speaker	None.

Speech

Rate:	Intelligibility:	Prosody:	Articulation:	Fluency:
WFL	WFL in known and unknown contexts; however, moderate-severe vocal hoarseness noted.	WFL	No articulation errors	WFL

Auditory Comprehension

Answering Yes/No Questions:	Executing Commands:	Understanding Stories & Paragraphs:	Understanding Conversational Speech:	Identifying Objects & their Functions:
WFL for concrete and personal yes/no questions; moderate-severe impairment at the abstract level.	Execution of one-step commands was WFL. Following complex, multi-step directions was moderately impaired.	Moderately impaired for stories comprised of three or more events.	Variable depending on complexity of information.	WFL

Reading

Word-level Comprehension:	Sentence-level Comprehension:	Oral Reading:	Oral Spelling:
WFL	Able to read the daily newspaper and understand its basic contents.	WFL for his pre-morbid educational level.	WFL for regularly spelled words.

Written Expression

Copying:	Writing to Dictation:	Self-generated:	Written Spelling:	Drawing:
Able to copy words and sentences.	WFL up to sentence level.	Able to generate a list of shopping items and write basic sentences.	WFL for ADL needs.	Patient refused to complete this task.

Cognition

Attention/Concentration:	Visuospatial Skills:	Memory:	Executive Functions:
Variable; better when interested in topic, e.g., the War in Vietnam.	Geographic disorientation and unable to find his way back to his room independently.	Procedural memory intact for ADLs including minor home repairs and self-care; moderately impaired episodic memory requiring mnemonic devices.	Judgment and reasoning for home and public safety are compromised making him unsafe to live independently. Requires 24 hour supervision. Unable to plan his daily routine.

Behavioral Symptoms

Alertness:	Deficit awareness:	Frustration:	Emotional Lability:	Current Personality Characteristics:
Reduced level of alertness interferes with response accuracy.	Poor; anosagnosia; "There's nothing wrong with me, it's you people".	Agitated and aggressive; requires wrist restraints when out of bed (OOB) to chair.	Cries out of context.	Impulsive; angry at times due to dependency on others.

Figure 9–1. Diagnostic profile of Tommy.

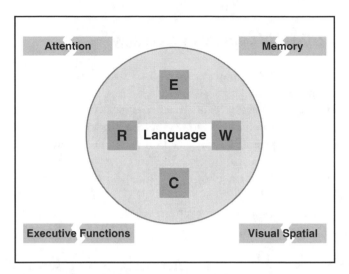

Figure 9–2. ALD Target Model for Tommy.

however, was functional for his ADL needs, although his ability to create a cohesive narrative discourse was inhibited. This was further complicated by Tommy's difficulty with turn-taking, impulsive responding characterized by interrupting the speaker, and inappropriate pause times. For example, if Tommy wanted to describe a special event he attended or relate information about his vacation experiences, the listener would need patience and understanding of Tommy's expressive language difficulties. Tommy's family/caregivers could use the training that they received from the SLP during his hospital stay to alert listeners to Tommy's expressive problems and cue him during his discourse and social interactions. Fortunately, Tommy demonstrated no lexical retrieval problems or paraphasias subsequent to his brain insult which is a good prognosticator for his eventual community re-entry. Tommy's speech intelligibility was 100% in known and unknown contexts and this was certainly to his benefit socially.

Tommy's procedural memory was intact for doing simple chores around the house and engaging in basic self-grooming tasks. However, his impaired episodic memory caused frustration and the family will need to use memory logs and daily personal logs to optimize his ability to function in his home and neighborhood environment. He is not safe to be left alone at this time. His judgment and reasoning for home and public safety scenarios were compromised. Consequently, Tommy needs 24-hour supervision at home until he begins to show progress in executive functioning. His anosagnosia (lack of deficit awareness) also complicates the home and public safety situation. He believed that he had no difficulty managing his daily routines and saw no need for close monitoring.

The SLP should recommend continued therapy at home once Tommy is discharged form the hospital. The SLP who treats Tommy at home, should continue to focus on deficit awareness, memory, family/counseling and education, and thought organization. Independent re-entry into the community may not be possible for him in the near future.

Critical Thinking/Learning Activity

- What is the speech-language pathologist's role in the evaluation of this type of patient?
- Based on Tommy's PMH is this an acute onset type or a progressive type of encephalopathy and what would be its etiology?
- How would this patient's lack of deficit awareness affect his ability to return to the social fabric of his environment?
- What are the family counseling and education issues in this case, and how would you address them?
- As an SLP, what characteristics would you look for to help differentiate the person with dementia and the person with a toxic-metabolic encephalopathy?
- What referrals would you make after assessing this case Why?

Treatment Considerations

Tommy's medical diagnosis was alcohol poisoning. Testing conducted over three sessions (due to patient's medical condition) revealed moderate cognitive-linguistic deficits. Tommy's auditory comprehension for simple, concrete information at the time of testing was WFL. However, due to his difficulty with more complex information presented auditorily, some environmental adjustments are necessary. For example, limiting the ambient noise, and limiting his communication partner to one person at a time are suggested. His family will need ongoing communication counseling while he is an inpatient and during his rehab stay since his auditory comprehension will affect his social interactions. Furthermore, his lack of deficit awareness, should it persist and become chronic, will complicate matters. Although Tommy's expressive language is functional for his ADL (activities of daily living) needs, it is mildly impaired. His greater deficits are in the cognitive areas of memory, thought organization, judgment, and reasoning. Consequently, Tommy will need to be supervised at home for compliance with his medications, appointments, and daily activities requiring organizational skills until he demonstrates the ability to manage these tasks independently and in sobriety. Drug and alcohol treatment is recommended for Tommy and his family.

It is important to remember the role that level of severity plays in the treatment planning and implementation for patients with encephalopathy. Furthermore, intervention is always provided within a functional/compensatory framework in these cases, and not one of remediation. The speech-language pathologist should consider the following treatment approaches when planning therapy for people with encephalopathy of any of the above mentioned types:

- When working with this type of patient, it is important to provide family/caregiver counseling and education, which are critical elements to the rehabilitation of the patient with encephalopathy. The family/caregivers need to understand: the cause of the encephalopathy, the results of the cognitive-linguistic evaluation, the goals of therapeutic intervention, and how to communicate effectively with this type of patient. For example, it is best not to expect the patient to do things that he or she cannot understand or execute successfully, and calling attention to their deficits is often unproductive. Instead, instruct the family/caregivers to support the patient by implementing the compensatory strategies at home that were developed during his stay at the hospital or rehab facility. Providing them with written information will help to reinforce therapeutic objectives and eliminate any misinterpretation of the verbally presented information.

■ Memory books and daily logs can be used to optimize the patient's ability to perform his/her ADLs. The clinician facilitates the patient's completion of the daily log and discusses the content. Developing activities to facilitate spatial and temporal orientation are also helpful with these patients.

■ Cotreating with occupational therapy and/or therapeutic recreation personnel provides the ability to integrate aspects of the patient's premorbid life into his life postonset. Furthermore, it provides a context within which to optimize the patient's social language, and to incorporate his or her behavioral goals as well. Working in a group promotes generalization of skills developed during individual therapy.

■ The clinician should consider consulting the Office of Vocational Rehabilitation (OVR) to determine if the patient's skill set post-therapy would support employment. The speech-language pathologist can then work with the OVR representative to enhance and/or reinforce the skills needed for a particular job.

Some Therapeutic Options

■ Therapeutic approaches addressing cognitive-communicative impairment (Helm-Estabrooks, 1995).

■ Graphic and written cues may be used to provide written information and photos to support recognition memory. Use of a memory wallet, book, or daily log is also suggested (Hoerster, Hickey, & Bourgeois, 2001).

■ Montessori-based interventions help to create structured and stimulating activities for social interaction (Orsulic-Jeras, Schneider, & Camp, 2001).

■ Spaced Retrieval Training (SRT) is a verbally mediated memory technique that may be used to develop safety awareness and support activities of daily living. The patient rehearses a specific response or action to a stimulus across repeated trials. The time between the presentation of the stimulus and the request from the clinician for the response are gradually increased. The patient eventually learns the new behavior. For example, writing one's name requires certain steps to accomplish

the act. The SLP may use Spaced Retrieval Training to facilitate the learning of these steps (Camp, Foss, O'Hanlon, & Stevens, 1996).
■ Additional therapeutic materials may include memory books and daily logs to assist with spatial and temporal orientation as well as planning, organizing and implementing daily routines. Also, board games and card games can be used to develop attentional skills and facilitate focus and concentration.

References

Camp, C. J., Foss, J. W., O'Hanlon, A. M., & Stevens, A. B. (1996). Memory intervention for persons with dementia. *Applied Cognitive Psychology, 10,* 193–210.

Helm-Estabrooks, N. (1995). *Cognitive-linguistic task book.* Sandwich, MA: Cape Cod Institute.

Hoerster, L., Hickey, E., & Bourgeois, M. (2001). Effects of memory aids on conversations between nursing home residents with dementia and nursing assistants. *Neuropsychological Rehabilitation, 11*(3 & 4), 399–427.

NINDS, National Institute of Neurological Disorders and Stroke. (2007). *NINDS Encephalopathy Information Page.* Retrieved September 8, 2008, from http://www.ninds.nih.gov/disorders/encephalopathy/encephalopathy.htm

Orsulic-Jeras, S., Schneider, N. M., & Camp, C. J., et al. (2001). Montessori-based dementia activities in long-term care: Training and implementation. *Activities, Adaptation, and Aging, 25,* 107–120.

Shulman, L. M., & Romano, J. G. (1999). Neurologic emergencies. In William J. Weiner & Christopher G. Goetz (Eds.), *Neurology for the non-neurologist* (4th ed., pp. 407–430). Philadelphia: Lipppincott Williams and Wilkins.

Substance Abuse and Mental Health Services Administration, Office of Applied Studies. (2006). *Results from the 2005 national survey on drug use health: National findings* (NSDUH Series H-30, DHHS Publication No. SMA-06-4194) (Table G.29). Rockville, MD: Author.

Chapter 10

REVIEW OF TREATMENT IN ACQUIRED LANGUAGE DISORDERS: PAST, PRESENT, AND FUTURE CONSIDERATIONS

Historical Overview of Efficacy and Evidence in the Treatment of ALD in Adults

Any discussion regarding the treatment efficacy in acquired language disorders in adults, and specifically, aphasia rehabilitation, must begin with Darley's 1972 paper on the topic (Darley, 1972). Although our book has discussed various acquired language disorders in adults, we believe that using Darley as a platform to discuss treatment efficacy is an appropriate starting place due to his generalizable reasoning. Darley found 10 "reports" that were mostly descriptive analyses and retrospective in nature. He concluded that the data were not robust and that any clinician must be cautious when making statements about treatment efficacy. Darley's article is seminal and the reader is directed to Wertz and Irwin's thorough, clear, and concise synopsis of it (Wertz & Irvin, 2001).

Darley proposed three general questions which the clinician must confront and answer in order to determine if the treatment protocols used in aphasia rehabilitation are effective (Darley, 1972, pp. 4–5):

1. Does language rehabilitation accomplish measureable gains in language function beyond what can be expected to occur as a result of spontaneous recovery?

2. Are the language gains attributable to therapy worth the necessary investment of time, effort, and money?

3. What are the relative degrees of effectiveness of various modes of treatment of aphasia?

Furthermore, Darley also offered four "fundamental considerations" that one must address in the design of any efficacy studies of treatment in aphasia (Darley, 1972):

1. The patients in a study of treatment in aphasia must be aphasic. Darley was not convinced that the descriptions of the aphasic syndromes existing at the time of his writing were accurate. Furthermore he admonished researchers to recognize and thoroughly describe any concomitant conditions, for example, apraxia of speech, confusion, and so forth.

2. There must be a clear differentiation between improvement based on therapeutic intervention and spontaneous recovery, which requires control subjects who are not included in the therapy program. This raises the ethical question of denying treatment to those in need, but for a study to be rigorous and valid this is the best experimental scenario.

3. In order to monitor change, the clinician must gather quantitative data that are reliable and objective. More interesting in today's context of

functionality, is Darley's interest in monitoring changes in the patient's behavior and quality of life by measuring psychological and psychosocial status before and after therapy. He even suggested using evoked potentials to make these measurements.

4. The clinician must clearly define and describe the procedures followed, the rationale, and the materials employed and that therapy must be delivered by "trained professionals" (Darley, 1972, p.14).

As noted above, Darley considered that the data at his time of writing was sparse and unconvincing. Returning to his three questions, the following information has emerged:

1. *Does language rehabilitation accomplish measureable gains in language function beyond what can be expected to occur as a result of spontaneous recovery?*
   It apparently does. Robey (1998) conducted a meta-analysis of efficacy studies in aphasia treatment and found that those patients who received treatment had better long-term outcomes than those who were not treated. This included patients at all stages of their recovery. Robey's work in this area is an important follow-up to Darley's and the clinician should become familiar with it. The reader is directed to Robey (1994) and Robey (1998).

2. *Are the language gains attributable to therapy worth the necessary investment of time, effort, and money?*
   There are no current data to answer this question. Researchers however, have addressed the issue of cost versus benefit, but arrived at no firm conclusions (Brookshire, 1994; Shewan & Kertesz, 1984; Wertz et al., 1986). How does one measure the cost of treatment versus nontreatment in a realistic way? The researchers above attempted to do so by calculating the cost per increase in scores on a language test or percentile rank. However, a truer cost/benefit analysis must measure changes in *functionality*. Is the patient now able to communicate effectively in a social context? Has the patient's quality of life improved as a result of language rehabilitation? Has there

been a reduction in the language deficits subsequent to language intervention? Wertz and Irwin (2001) suggest that perhaps we should be measuring whether the patient's improvement can be noticed by a "naive observer" (p. 244). Obviously, this is a critical question requiring a serious answer from the discipline as it has therapeutic and sociopolitical implications.

3. *What are the relative degrees of effectiveness of various modes of treatment of aphasia?*
   The current answer to this question is that there does not seem to be any significant differences between the different treatment approaches used in aphasia. Wertz et al. (1981) did report that there was a small but significant difference in the outcomes of patients who were treated individually versus those treated in a group setting. However, more recent work with adults in groups within the LPAA context has shown efficacy (Elman & Bernstein-Ellis, 1999).

Randomized Controlled Trials (RCTs) and Aphasia Treatment

Greener, Enderby, and Whurr (1999) stimulated vigorous discussion among speech-language pathologists when they concluded that aphasia treatment had not been shown to be "clearly effective or clearly ineffective within a randomized controlled trial (RCT)" (p. 1). In typical experiments, subjects are assigned to groups randomly. However, in the case of studies conducted with aphasic individuals, presence in a group is determined by the presence and type of aphasia and are considered quasiexperiments (Douglas et al., 2002). Robey (1998) identified 479 studies and found 55 quasiexperiments in his meta-analysis. One of the interesting findings Robey reported was that there was actually a decrease in the number of RCTs conducted since the 1980s. Despite this, he did report the following findings from his meta-analysis:

1. The patients who were treated had better outcomes than those who did not have treatment in all stages of recovery across time postonset.
2. The patient outcome was better when treatment was started in the acute phase of recovery.

3. Patients who received greater than 2 hours of therapy per week had better outcomes than those who received less.

4. The most commonly reported form of treatment was individual.

5. The largest gains were seen in those patients who were rated as severe and moderately-severe. No study in his analysis was designed to measure treatment effects in the mildly impaired patient population.

6. There were not enough studies examining the differential effects for the different types of aphasia therapy, for example, Melodic Intonation Therapy versus Stimulation-Facilitation Therapy.

Although the results on efficacy in this analysis were not as powerful as one would hope, the support for intervention at all levels of recovery is worth noting. Of the 12 studies reported on by Greener et al. (1999), only one used an RCT design. It appears that this move away from RCTs is related to the emergence of the single subject design which motivated Robey et al. (1999) to conduct a meta-analysis of research on the efficacy of single-subject experiments in aphasia treatment. Unfortunately, only 12 out of 63 single-subject studies that Robey and his colleagues reported on provided quantifiable results (Robey, 1999). The authors found this unsatisfactory concluding that single-subject designs were not able to produce evidence that supported the effectiveness of any given treatment (Robey, 1998).

The obvious challenges for researchers interested in using RCTs in aphasiology or any brain disorder are the issues of patient variability, selection criteria, well-described treatment protocols, objective and quantifiable results, and ethical considerations. As can be seen from the above discussion, RCTs in communication sciences and disorders have not been forthcoming. If, however, the single-subject design is the preferred methodology for testing the efficacy of treatment in communication sciences and disorders, then there needs to be rigorous protocols in place that allow for replication, multiple baselines, and produce results for functional outcomes. That is, future research into treatment efficacy must find a way to measure quality of life issues in the aphasic population as well as changes in test results, and so forth, post-treatment. Thus, this is a call for single-

subject, and for that matter any group designs, to include both quantitative and qualitative measures so that efficacy can be determined in functional and objective domains.

We believe that Darley (1972) "hit the nail on the head." His questions have not been satisfactorily answered and his "fundamental considerations" are powerfully relevant today. If we keep his mandate in mind as we continue to critically examine our practice, we believe that we will eventually arrive at the desired outcome: finding the best cost/time effective approaches that hold the welfare of the patient paramount while providing functional benefits to the patient within his social milieu.

Treatment Approaches and Future Trends

Research in the treatment of adults with acquired language disorders is advancing. Recent reviews have focused on three exciting avenues of intervention. These interventions reflect advances in biological/pharmacologic knowledge, research about intensity of treatment, and changes based on computer-assisted technologies that are cost-effective and time efficient. All of these point to a future of growth for us as clinicians and enhanced outcomes for our patients. We address each of these briefly below.

Biological and Pharmacologic Interventions

The advent of pharmacologic interventions to increase blood flow in the acute phase of stroke, combined with new discoveries about neuroplasticity in the adult and the possibility of infusing the brain with new tissue all contribute to a future of great promise for the rehabilitation of the stroke patient with language disorder. Wineburgh and Small (2004) propose that the treatment of aphasia in the adult is at a crossroads where all three of the above-mentioned variables can come together to improve language rehabilitation outcomes. However, these biological aspects of intervention must be supplemented with and complemented by behavioral therapy, that is, speech-language therapies in order for the person with aphasia to integrate the benefits of the biological changes into their daily behaviors.

The current practices in treatment of aphasia have been shown to be effective (Robey, 1998). However, looking toward the future, Wineburgh and Small (2004) believe that in cases where biological intervention occurs, for example, stem cell infusion or neuronal implantation, the speech-language pathologist will be required to determine if his intervention is "harmful" or "beneficial" to the patient after the procedure. As we know very little about the biology of language processes, the clinician will need to understand if the speech-language intervention *postprocedure* will facilitate recovery or inhibit it. This requires a shift in thinking from "effective" therapy to "beneficial" therapy (Wineburgh & Small, 2004). Our current practice does not include biological intervention; however, with the emergence of stem cell technology and more refined knowledge of cortical neurophysiology poststroke, the speech-language pathologist can look forward to a very exciting future in which she will play a major role in the functional rehabilitation of the adult with an acquired language disorder.

There is a long history of using pharmacologic agents in the treatment of aphasia, starting with Alexander Luria, the Soviet neurologist, who used galanthamine (an anticholinesterase agent) to improve speech, language, cognitive and motor functions in people with stroke (Webb & Adler, 2008). Other drugs used in the treatment of aphasia include bromocriptine (dopaminergic), amphetamines, cholinergic agents, GABAergic agents, and serotoninergic agents. Berthier (2005), reported that pharmacologic agents that act on the catecholamine system, for example, bromocriptine, have demonstrated variable results in the treatment of people with aphasia in placebo-controlled studies. The findings on bromocriptine, however, show very selective effectiveness. It appears that it is most effective in acute and chronic aphasia of the nonfluent type and in cases of reduced verbal initiation, for example, transcortical motor aphasia (Berthier, 2005). Donepizil, a drug acting on the cholinergic system, showed more promise in chronic aphasias, was well tolerated by the patients, and its efficacy was maintained over the

long term (Berthier, 2005). Although Wineburgh and Small (2004) report that pharmacotherapy "has never been shown to have any effectiveness" in the treatment of aphasia, Webb and Adler (2008) point out that pharmacologic intervention seem to be useful complements to traditional treatment approaches to aphasia. The controversy continues but as biochemical technology advances and the pathophysiology of stroke continues to be refined, expect to see more agents coming onto the market for the treatment of aphasia.

Intensity of Treatment

Current fiscal constraints, imposed by CMS (Center for Medicare and Medicaid Services) and private insurers on rehabilitation services, restrict the duration of speech-language pathology services available to people with aphasia. Therefore, it makes good clinical and fiscal sense, within the context of health care today, to provide the best service and to obtain the best outcome in the shortest amount of time. In a meta-analysis conducted by Robey (1998) he concluded that providing at least 2 hours of therapy per week facilitated gains in patients and recommended that two hours per week should constitute a minimum of therapeutic services for people with aphasia. Bhogal et al. (2003) also conducted a metanalysis of studies investigating aphasia therapy, and found that a significant treatment effect followed 8.8 hours of therapy per week for 11.2 weeks versus studies that provided only 2 hours of therapy per week for 22.9 weeks. They concluded that speech outcomes are clearly improved if an intensive schedule of therapy is used in patients with aphasia.

The Rehabilitation Institute of Chicago (RIC) is leading the way in the area of intensive therapy for people with aphasia. Their program—The RIC Intensive Therapy Aphasia Program—provides daily, individual therapy for two hours per day; one hour of computer-based treatment; two hours of group therapy targeting reading, writing, and conversational skills; one hour of more specialized treatment with programs such as PACE or AAC devices; and caregiver workshops and support. This offers the patient a total of approximately 30 hours of therapy per week for 4 weeks. These programs were developed at RIC; in order to be eligible, a patient must be at least 18 years old, medically stable, must be able to tolerate the intensity of the therapy, and be either independent in mobility and self-care or be accompanied by a caregiver at all times (Rehabilitation Institute of Chicago, 2008).

Computer-Assisted Technology and Treatment of Aphasia

Katz (2008) defines computerized aphasia treatment as the "systematic use of computers and software to improve communication skills in people with aphasia" (p. 852). The straightforwardness of the definition, however, cloaks the complexity of the issue. Katz states that there are three roles that computer-only treatment (COT) and computer-assisted treatment (CAT) play in aphasia therapy:

1. COT programs allow the patient to practice independent of the clinician, family, and/or caregiver once the clinician has designed the treatment program for that patient. This type of software program usually consists of drills.
2. CAT software programs allow the patient and the clinician to work side-by-side. The role of the computer is to present the material whereas the role of the patient and clinician was a dynamic and interactive one using the software program as the therapy material.
3. Alternative and augmentative communication (AAC) in aphasia therapy refers to computers that can utilize icons, digitized speech, animation, and are used to facilitate functional communication for the person with aphasia.

The clinician is not accustomed to working within a therapeutic context that does not necessarily include the familiar framework of delivering the treatment, measuring the patient's performance, modifying the treatment, and then treating with the modified version. Yet, within the CAT, COT, and AAC paradigm this more conventional approach to rehabilitation is not always possible, nor appropriate. Consequently, Katz (2008) summarizes three models of rehabilitation that are applicable when using computers in aphasia therapy.

Brain-Behavior Relationships

Essentially, this model adheres to the philosophy that language rehabilitation can happen through retraining and works on the premise that the patient can regain lost skills through reorganizing the brain functions that have been damaged.

Behavior Modification

Operant conditioning achieves behavior modification by systematically applying consequences after a stimulus is given. The organism can learn a new behavior or lose an old one. Computer programs can provide a stimulus and reinforce the patient for a correct response, through feedback.

Educational Models

These programs can create "microworlds" within which the patient can "operate" and learn to solve problems associated with their daily communication needs. The type of learning in this case is not didactic but more inductive. The patient can discover the answers as opposed to being told the answers. Games designed to facilitate rehabilitation of functional language skills certainly have a place in the repertoire of any clinician using CAT and COT methodology.

Within any of these models, the clinician can decide to use stimulation, simulation, drills or tutorials as treatment protocols since all four of these are available and possible with computer software programs today (Katz, 2008).

Lee and Cherney (2008) describe an interactive computer software program called AphasiaScripts™, developed at RIC, which provides both intensive therapy and computer-assisted approaches to treatment. The program is designed to allow the patient to gain practice in conversation. In this approach, an avatar acts as the virtual clinician, that is, conversational partner. The authors describe the program as user-friendly for the patient, but it still requires the expertise of a speech-language pathologist to facilitate the patient's ability to interact with the program. For example, the patient, with the assistance of the clinician, learns how to use cueing to optimize performance so that he can practice the conversations intensively without a clinician present. AphasiaScripts™ incorporates both intensity of treatment and the use of computer-assisted technology in order to optimize patient outcomes.

The crucial link in the therapeutic chain between the patient and any CAT, COT, or AAC methods is the speech-language pathologist. It is the clinician who evaluates the patient, designs the treatment objectives, determines which tasks are to be used to implement those objectives and then trains the patient to use the device or program. That is, there is an "intelligent division of labor between computers and clinician" and the boundaries are clear (Katz, 2008, p. 869). The fine nuances of human interaction cannot be overstated, especially within the context of a therapeutic interaction. CAT and COT technology promises to broaden a clinician's treatment options and optimize patient progress.

Constraint-Induced Language Therapy (CILT)

Constraint-induced therapy, developed from animal research, is modeled after treatment used in physical therapy (Cherney, Patterson, Raymer, Frymark, & Schooling, 2008). This technique was introduced in 2001 and is primarily used with patients with nonfluent aphasia (Cherney et al., 2008). It is based on three principles: massed practice, constraint induction, and behavioral relevance (Pulvermuller et al., 2001). The mechanism responsible for the success of this therapy is currently unknown. However, the mechanism seems to be related to the way motor constraint overcomes learned non-use (Pulvermuller et al., 2001). Regarding language, learned non-use may result from the individual's failure to produce complex verbal utterances and the reinforcement the patient gets from the therapist when he or she uses an alternative communication method to convey meaning.

There have been positive effects from this treatment approach particularly due to its high intensity. Unlike traditional approaches in aphasia therapy that focus on compensatory strategies such as drawing and writing, this approach requires only attempts at verbal communication, which is the "induced constraint." It is recommended that patients receive the maximum of 3 hours of therapy per day, five days

per week. In this approach the therapist presents the patient with tasks that require him or her to name objects pictured on cards, such as a card picturing a muffin. The patient is required to name the item using the correct noun, and as they progress the clinician adds a modifier, for example, two muffins. As they became more advanced they must put that phrase into a syntactic frame, using the name of the person they are addressing, for example, "Mrs. Jones, can I please have two muffins?" Research indicates that patients who received CILT had a 30% increase in the amount of daily verbal communication used, as reported on their Communication Activity Logs (CAL) (Pulvermuller et al., 2001). It is speculated that there may be cortical reorganization from massed practice that promotes language rehabilitation. Cherney et al. (2008) found that regardless of treatment type, more treatment appears to produce better results when delivered over a restricted time period. Regardless of the treatment approach used, clinicians must make treatment decisions based on clinical experience, the patient's individualized needs, and sound evidence of treatment efficacy.

The Use of Video Games in the Rehabilitation of the ALD Patient

Physical and occupational therapists have been using video gaming to assist with the arm and hand rehabilitation of their patients (Adriaenssens, Eggermont, Pyck, Boeckx, & Gilles, 1988; King, 1993; Szer, 1983). Although computerized programs are used in the rehabilitation of adults with communication disorders, there is no mention in the literature about the use of video gaming as a possible tool for rehabilitation. We believe that the clinician may want to consider this approach for patients presenting with cognitive impairment. More specifically, gaming matches perfectly the needs of patients like Debra—those with right hemispheric impairments and TBI patients like Samuel. Consequently, we suggest that the clinician may want to consider video gaming to facilitate growth in the following areas:

- Memory
- Thought organization
- Planning

- Visuospatial skills
- Visual scanning
- Attention to task

Patients with aphasia also may benefit. For example, using the game as a platform for building a narrative, lexical retrieval, and for sentence building are possible uses. We suggest that the clinician supplements more traditional programs that do have proven efficacy with gaming, since there are no efficacy studies for this approach. Games would need to be selected based on type of disorder, severity of disorder, age of client, content, and applicability, which are essentially the same criteria the clinician would use to assess more traditional programs for his or her patient. For example, there are a number of simulation games that use animals, people, towns, and more. These games allow the user to create life events, stories, and engage in problem-solving behavior with outcomes that affect their characters. One example of this type of game is The Sims (http://www.thesims3.com).

It is important to remember that returning the patient to a functional communication status is always the ultimate goal of any treatment approach in ALD. In today's health care environment, with the constraints on reimbursement and number of visits permitted by insurers, the clinician must think creatively and innovatively to meet the long-term goal of functional communication.

For a review of Selected Treatment Programs and Approaches, see Appendix E.

References

Adriaenssens, E., Eggermont, E., Pyck, K., Boeckx, W., & Gilles, B. (1988). The video invasion of rehabilitation. *Burns, 14*, 417-419.

Berthier, M. L. (2005). Postroke aphasia: Epidemiology, pathophysiology and treatment. *Drugs and Aging, 22*(2), 163-182.

Bhogal, S. K., Teasell, R., & Speechley, M. (2003). Intensity of aphasia therapy, impact on recovery. *Stroke, 34*, 987.

Brookshire, R. H. (1994). Group studies of treatment for adults with aphasia: Efficacy, effectiveness and believability. *ASHA Special Interest Divisions: Neurophysiology and Neurogenic Speech and Language Disorders, 4*, 5-13.

Cherney, L. R., Patterson, J. P., Raymer, A., Frymark, T., & Schooling, T. (2008). Evidence-based systematic review: Effects of intensity of treatment and constraint-induced language therapy for individuals with stroke-induced aphasia. *Journal of Speech, Language, and Hearing Research, 51*, 1282-1289.

Darley, F. L. (1972). The efficacy of language rehabilitation in aphasia. *Journal of Speech and Hearing Disorders, 37*, 3-21.

Douglas, J., Brown, L., & Barry, S. (2002). Is aphasia therapy effective? Exploring the evidence in systematic reviews. *Brain Impairment, 3*(1), 17-27.

Elman, R., & Bernstein-Ellis, E. (1999). The efficacy of group communication treatment in adults with chronic aphasia. *Journal of Speech, Language, and Hearing Research, 42*, 411-419.

Greener, J., Enderby, P., & Whurr, R. (1999). Speech and language therapy for aphasia following stroke (Cochrane Review). In *The Cochrane Library, Issue 4* (Dec), Oxford: BMJ Books/Update Software.

Katz, R. (2008). Computer applications in aphasia treatment. In R. Chapey (Ed.), *Language intervention strategies in aphasia and related neurogenic communication disorders* (5th ed., pp. 852-876). Philadelphia: Lippincott Williams & Wilkins.

King, T. (1993). Hand strengthening with a computer for purposeful activity. *American Journal of Occupational Therapy, 47*, 635-637.

Lee, J. B., & Cherney, L. R. (2008). The changing "face" of aphasia. *Perspectives on Neurophysiology and Neurogenic Speech and Language Disorders, 18*, 15-23.

Pulvermuller, F., Neininger, B., Elbert, T., Mohr, B., Rockstroh, B., Koebbel, P., et al. (2001). Constraint-induced therapy of chronic aphasia after stroke. *Stroke, 32*, 1621-1626.

Rehabilitation Institute of Chicago. (2008). *RIC offers new intensive aphasia therapy program.* Retrieved August 11, 2008, from http://www.ric.org/aboutus/mediacenter/press/2008/07012008.aspx

Robey, R. R. (1994). The efficacy of treatment of aphasic persons: A meta-analysis. *Brain and Language, 47*, 582-608.

Robey, R. R. (1998). A metanalysis of clinical outcomes in the treatment of aphasia. *Journal of Speech and Hearing Research, 41*, 172-187.

Robey, R., Schultz, M., Crawford, A., & Sinner, C. (1999). Single-subject clinical outcome research: Design, data, effect sizes, and analyses. *Aphasiology, 13*, 445-473.

Shewan, C., & Kertesz, A. (1984). Effects of speech language treatment in recovery from aphasia. *Brain and Language, 23,* 272–299.

Szer, J. (1983). Video games as physiotherapy. *Medical Journal of Australia, 1,* 401–402.

Webb, W. G., & Adler, R. K. (2008). *Neurology for the speech-language pathologist* (p. 243). Philadelphia: Elsevier.

Wertz, R. T., Collins, M. J., Weiss, D., Kurtzke, J. F., Friden, T., Brookshire, R. H., et al. (1981). Veterans Administration cooperative study on aphasia: A comparison of individual and group treatment. *Journal of Speech and Hearing Research, 24,* 580–594.

Wertz, R. T., & Irwin, W. H. (2001). Darley and the efficacy of language rehabilitation in aphasia. *Aphasiology, 15*(3), 231–247.

Wertz, R. T., Weiss, D. G., Aten, J. L., Brookshire, R. H., Garcia-Bunuel, L., Holland, A. L., et al. (1986). Comparison of clinic, home, and deferred language treatment for aphasia. A Veterans Administration Cooperative Study. *Archives of Neurology, 43,* 653–658.

Wineburgh, L. F., & Small, S. L. (2004, April 27). Aphasia treatment and the crossroads: A biological perspective. *The ASHA Leader,* pp. 6–7, 18.

Appendix A

SPEECH-LANGUAGE PATHOLOGY CASE HISTORY FORM

Name: _____ Age: _____ Date: _____

Reason for Admission

_____

_____

_____

_____

Past Medical History

_____

_____

_____

_____

_____

Psychosocial History (Occupation, home environment, etc.)

_____

_____

_____

_____

_____

Consults (Service and Findings)

_____

_____

_____

_____

_____

Imaging Study Results (CT, MRI, Angiography, etc.)

_____

_____

_____

_____

Other Relevant Test Results

_____

_____

_____

Relevant Lab Results

_____

_____

_____

Family/Caregiver Contact Information

_____

_____

_____

_____

Appendix B

SKILLS ASSESSMENT INVENTORY

The Skills Assessment Inventory (SAI) is to be used by the clinician and the client's family to help identify functional therapeutic activities prior to treatment.

How to Use the SAI

To assess each skill, observe the client, ask for his or her input when possible, and obtain information from family members or close friends to determine those skills that you will target in treatment. Circle the number from 0 to 5 that best corresponds with the clients perceived ability to perform each task. Items scored in the middle ability range (3s and 4s) should be targeted first because they will allow the client to experience some success. Those that are rated as difficult (0s and 1s) should be avoided initially; they may present frustration. Once you have targeted a few important skills that are in the middle ability level, turn to the corresponding activity pages in this manual and follow the specified directions. Monitor progress on an ongoing basis. We suggest you revisit the client's SAI on a monthly basis.

Note. It is not essential that the client work on all activities in this manual. Select those that relate to the client's life and personal needs. From E. R. Klein & S. E. Hahn, *Focus on Function: Graining Essential Communication, 2nd edition*, 2007, Pro-Ed. Reprinted with permission.

0 = Not applicable	2 = Much difficulty in performing task	4 = Usually independent
1 = Unable to perform	3 = Performs task with assistance	5 = Normal functioning

PART I: Basic Living Skills

Chapter 1 Basic Communications						
1. Expressing Needs and Desires	0	1	2	3	4	5
2. Starting Conversations	0	1	2	3	4	5
3. Responding to Emergency and Safety Situations	0	1	2	3	4	5
4. Understanding Common Phrases	0	1	2	3	4	5
5. Talking to Service Personnel	0	1	2	3	4	5
Chapter 2 Using a Telephone						
6. Using a Phone	0	1	2	3	4	5
7. Using a Telephone Directory	0	1	2	3	4	5
8. Using a Phone to Call for Assistance	0	1	2	3	4	5
9. Making Appointments	0	1	2	3	4	5
10. Using the Phone to Get Information	0	1	2	3	4	5
11. Taking Phone Messages	0	1	2	3	4	5
Chapter 3 Managing and Understanding Time						
12. Understanding Measurements of Time	0	1	2	3	4	5
13. Setting a Clock and Telling Time	0	1	2	3	4	5
14. Designing a Daily Schedule	0	1	2	3	4	5
15. Designing a Weekly Schedule	0	1	2	3	4	5
16. Following Calendar Dates and Appointments	0	1	2	3	4	5
17. Recording Events and Keeping a Log	0	1	2	3	4	5
Chapter 4 Managing and Understanding Finances						
18. Understanding Basic Measurements of Money	0	1	2	3	4	5
19. Understanding Bills	0	1	2	3	4	5
20. Writing Checks and Balancing a Checkbook	0	1	2	3	4	5
21. Using an Automated Teller Machine (ATM)	0	1	2	3	4	5
22. Understanding Bank Statements	0	1	2	3	4	5
23. Understanding Graphs and Charts	0	1	2	3	4	5

Chapter 5 Shopping						
24. Working with Money to Purchase Items	0	1	2	3	4	5
25. Using Coupons and Calculating Discounts	0	1	2	3	4	5
Chapter 6 Meals and Cooking						
26. Understanding Basic Measurements and Quantity	0	1	2	3	4	5
27. Planning Menus and Writing Shopping Lists	0	1	2	3	4	5
28. Using Microwave Oven	0	1	2	3	4	5
29. Cooking with Recipes	0	1	2	3	4	5
Chapter 7 Getting Around						
30. Reading Signs and Symbols	0	1	2	3	4	5
31. Reading Maps	0	1	2	3	4	5
32. Giving Directions to Places	0	1	2	3	4	5
Chapter 8 Activities Around the House						
33. Understanding Measurements of Distance	0	1	2	3	4	5
34. Sequencing Daily Events	0	1	2	3	4	5
35. Reading Directions to Accomplish Tasks	0	1	2	3	4	5
36. Giving Directions to Complete Tasks	0	1	2	3	4	5
37. Using Math to Solve Common Problems	0	1	2	3	4	5
38. Filling in Order Forms	0	1	2	3	4	5
39. Ordering from a Catalog	0	1	2	3	4	5
40. Reading Automobile Classified Advertisements	0	1	2	3	4	5
41. Writing Classified Advertisements	0	1	2	3	4	5
42. Writing Letters	0	1	2	3	4	5
43. Addressing Envelopes	0	1	2	3	4	5

PART II: Social, Leisure, and Work Activities

Chapter 9 Social Participation						
44. Understanding Stories in Social Setting	0	1	2	3	4	5
45. Retelling Stories	0	1	2	3	4	5
46. Describing and Discussing Photos	0	1	2	3	4	5
47. Using Situational Speech in Dialogue	0	1	2	3	4	5

0 = Not applicable   2 = Much difficulty in performing task   4 = Usually independent

1 = Unable to perform   3 = Performs task with assistance   5 = Normal functioning

48. Performing Social Exchange	0	1	2	3	4	5
49. Expressing Opinions Through Dialogue	0	1	2	3	4	5
50. Discussing Feelings and Recognizing Emotions	0	1	2	3	4	5
51. Answering Questions Involving Quantity	0	1	2	3	4	5
52. Role Playing	0	1	2	3	4	5
53. Understanding Body Language and Facial Expression	0	1	2	3	4	5
54. Drawing Inferences from Photos	0	1	2	3	4	5
55. Understanding Idioms	0	1	2	3	4	5
Chapter 10 Leisure						
56. Finding Page Numbers	0	1	2	3	4	5
57. Reading Television and Cable Listings	0	1	2	3	4	5
58. Reading a Table of Contents	0	1	2	3	4	5
59. Understanding News Articles	0	1	2	3	4	5
60. Using a Dictionary	0	1	2	3	4	5
61. Understanding Restaurant Checks	0	1	2	3	4	5
62. Reading a Menu	0	1	2	3	4	5
63. Understanding Directions	0	1	2	3	4	5
64. Playing Games	0	1	2	3	4	5
65. Using the Internet	0	1	2	3	4	5
66. Communicating via Email	0	1	2	3	4	5
Chapter 11 Work						
67. Reading Help-Wanted Classified Advertisements	0	1	2	3	4	5
68. Completing Applications	0	1	2	3	4	5
69. Writing a Basic Résumé	0	1	2	3	4	5
70. Writing a Job Application Cover Letter	0	1	2	3	4	5
71. Creating a List of Professional and Personal References	0	1	2	3	4	5
72. Responding to Interview Questions	0	1	2	3	4	5
73. Solving Problems Through Dialogue	0	1	2	3	4	5

Appendix C

COGNITIVE LINGUISTIC EVALUATION

Name: _____ Age: _____ Date: _____

Primary Care Physician: _____

Medical Diagnosis: _____

Date of Incident: _____

Condition Prior to Incident: _____

Date of CT Scan/MRI: _____ Findings: _____

Relevant Medical History: _____

_____

_____

Medications: _____

Examiner: _____

Instructions: Administer selected sections or all sections as appropriate for the client. Specific instructions are provided under each subheading. Make additional observations in the right-hand column. The client will need a pen or pencil to complete the writing portion of the evaluation.

From K. G. Shipley & J. G. McAfee (2004). *Assessment in speech-language pathology: A resource manual* (3rd Ed.). Clifton Park, NY: Delmar Learning. Reprinted with permission.

Orientation and Awareness

Ask the client the following questions. Score a plus (+) or minus (−) for correct or incorrect responses.

Comments

____ What day is it?_____

____ What month is it? _____

____ What year is it? _____

____ What season is it? _____

____ Approximately what time do you think it is? _____

____ What state are we in? _____

____ What city are we in? _____

____ What county are we in?_____

____ Where do you live?_____

____ What is the name of this building?_____

____ Why are you in the hospital?_____

____ How long have you been here? _____

____ When did you have your accident? _____

____ What kind of problems do you have because of your accident?_____

____ What is my name? _____

____ What is my profession? _____

____ Who is your doctor?_____

____ About how much time has passed since we started talking together today? _____

Memory

Immediate Memory. Ask the client to repeat the following sequences or sentences. Score a plus (+) or minus (−) for correct or incorrect responses.

Comments

____ 0, 7, 4, 2 _____

____ 8, 6, 0, 1, 3 _____

____ 2, 9, 1, 4, 6, 5 _____

____ car, duck, ring, shoe _____

Comments

___ rain, desk, ladder, horse, cake _____

___ The keys were found under the table. _____

___ He always reads the newspaper before he has breakfast. _____

___ After their victory, the baseball team had pizza and watched a movie. _____

Ask the client to retell this story:

___ Helen had a birthday party at the petting zoo. Ten of her friends came. All the children laughed when a goat was found eating the cake and ice cream.

Recent memory. Ask the client the following questions. Score a plus (+) or minus (−) for correct or incorrect responses.

Comments

___ What did you have for breakfast? _____

___ What did you do after dinner last night? _____

___ What did you do after breakfast this morning? _____

___ What else have you done today? _____

___ Have you had any visitors today or yesterday? _____

___ What other therapies do you receive? _____

___ Who is your doctor? _____

___ How long have you been a resident here? _____

Long-term Memory. Ask the client the following questions. Score a plus (+) or a minus (-) for correct or incorrect responses.

Comments

___ Where were you born? _____

___ When is your birthday? _____

___ What is your husband's/wife's name? _____

___ How many children do you have? _____

___ How many grandchildren do you have? _____

___ Where did you used to work? _____

___ How much school did you complete? _____

___ Where did you grow up? _____

___ How many brothers and sisters do you have? _____

Auditory Processing and Comprehension

Ask the client the following questions. Score a plus (+) or minus (−) for correct or incorrect responses.

Comments

___ Is your last name Williams? _____

___ Is my name Jim? _____

___ Are you wearing glasses? _____

___ Do you live on the moon? _____

___ Have you had dinner yet? _____

___ Do cows eat grass? _____

___ Do fish swim? _____

___ Do four quarters equal one dollar? _____

___ Are there forty-eight hours in a day? _____

___ Is Alaska part of the United States?_____

Problem Solving

Ask the client the following questions. Score a plus (+) or minus (−) for correct or incorrect responses.

Comments

___ What would you do if you locked your keys in your house? _____

___ What would you do if your newspaper did not get delivered?_____

___ What would you do if you could not find your doctor's phone number? _____

___ What would you do if your TV stopped working? _____

___ What would you do if you forgot to put the milk away when you got home from the grocery store?

Logic, Reasoning, Inference

Ask the client what is wrong with these sentences. Score a plus (+) or minus (−) for correct or incorrect responses.

Comments

___ He put salt and pepper in his coffee._____

___ Six plus one is eight. _____

Comments

___ I put my socks on over my shoes. _____

___ Hang up when the phone rings._____

___ The dog had four kittens. _____

Ask the client what these expressions mean. Score a plus (+) or minus (−) for correct or incorrect responses.

Comments

___ Haste makes waste. _____

___ An apple a day keeps the doctor away. _____

___ When it rains it pours. _____

___ He's a chip off the old block. _____

___ Beauty is only skin deep. _____

Ask the client the following questions. Score a plus (+) or minus (−) for correct or incorrect responses.

Comments

___ What is worn on your feet, knit, and used to keep you warm? _____

___ What has a busy tail, climbs trees, and stores nuts? _____

___ What is thin and lightweight, used to wipe tears, and used during a cold? _____

___ How are a sweater, pants, and a blouse alike?_____

___ How are orange juice, soda, and milk alike? _____

Thought Organization

Ask the client to answer the following questions or tasks. Score a plus (+) or minus (−) for correct or incorrect responses.

Comments

___ What does the word "affectionate" mean? _____

___ What does the word "deliver" mean? _____

___ What are the steps you follow to wash your hair? _____

___ What are the steps you follow to make your bed? _____

___ How would you plan a meal for two dinner guests? _____

Calculation

Ask the client to answer the following questions. Score a plus (+) or minus (−) for correct or incorrect responses.

Comments

____ If you went to the mall and spent $8.00 in one store and $7.50 in another store, how much did you spend? _____

____ If tomatoes cost $1.50 per pound and you bought 2 pounds, how much did you spend on tomatoes? _____

____ If you went to the store with $3.00 and returned home with $1.75, how much did you spend? _____

____ If toothbrushes cost $3.00 each and you have $10.00, how many toothbrushes can you buy? _____

____ If you have a doctor's appointment at 10:30 and it takes you 30 minutes to get there, what time should you leave? _____

Reading and Visual Processing

Ask the client to read the six words in each row and cross out the one that does not belong. Score a plus (+) or minus (−) for correct or incorrect responses.

____ Cow   Apple   Carrot   Cheese   Banana   Oatmeal

____ Desk   Chair   Blue   Bed   Couch   Table

Ask the client to read the following sentences and do what they say. Score a plus (+) or minus (−) for correct or incorrect responses.

Comments

____ Look at the ceiling. _____

____ Point to the door, then blink your eyes. _____

____ Sing Happy Birthday. _____

Ask the client to read the following paragraph out loud and answer the questions about it. Score a plus (+) or minus (−) for correct or incorrect responses.

Mark and Rick are brothers. They both entered a tennis tournament, hoping to win the $1000 grand prize. Mark won his first two matches, but was eliminated after losing the third match. Rick made it all the way to the semi-finals. He lost, but was awarded a can of tennis balls as a consolation prize.

Comments

____ Are Mark and Rick cousins? _____

____ What sport did they play? _____

Comments

___ What was the grand prize? _____

___ Did one of them win the grand prize?_____

___ Which one did the best in the tournament? _____

Show the client these two clocks and ask them what time the clocks say. Score a plus (+) or minus (−) for correct or incorrect responses.

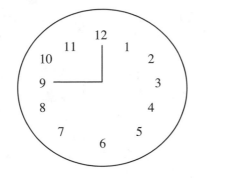 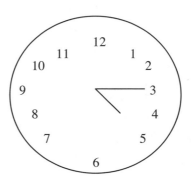

Now ask the client to copy the clocks below. Note accuracy of construction.

Ask the client to put an x through all the circles on this page. Note the client's attention to the left half of the page.

Write your name.

Write today's date.

Write a short description of what you have done today in speech therapy.

Writing

Ask the client to complete the writing tasks presented on the opposite page. Observe accuracy of response, completeness, and organization of response, legibility, and observance of left visual field. Make comments in the right margin.

Comments

Write your name. _____

Write today's date. _____

Write a short description of what you have done today in speech therapy. _____

_____

Pragmatics and Affect

Check all behaviors observed during your assessment.

Comments

____ Inappropriate physical proximity_____

____ Inappropriate physical contacts _____

____ Left visual field neglect _____

____ Poor eye contact_____

____ Lack of facial expression _____

____ Gestures (inappropriate, absent) _____

____ Lack of prosodic features of speech (intensity, pitch, rhythm) _____

____ Poor topic maintenance _____

____ Lack of appropriate turn taking _____

____ Perseveration _____

____ Presupposition (too much, too little) _____

____ Inappropriately verbose_____

____ Lack of initiation_____

____ Easily distracted _____

____ Frequent interruptions_____

____ Impulsive_____

____ Poor organization _____

____ Incompleteness _____

Appendix D

ACQUIRED LANGUAGE DISORDERS (ALD) TARGET MODELS

Appendix E

SELECTED TREATMENT PROGRAMS AND APPROACHES

Anagram, Copy, and Recall Therapy (ACRT)

Divergent Word Retrieval

High-Tech Alternative and Augmentative Communication (AAC) Devices

Lexical Retrieval and Sentence Production Programs

    Cueing Hierarchies

    Comprehension Tasks That Facilitate Oral Naming

    Semantic Feature Analysis

    Normal Sentence Production

    Mapping Treatment

    Treatment of Underlying Forms

    Melodic Intonation Therapy

Life Participation Approach to Aphasia (LPAA)

Melodic Intonation Therapy (MIT)

Narrative Story Cards

Nonsymbolic Movements for Activation of Intention (NMAI)

Promoting Aphasics' Communicative Effectiveness (PACE)

Response Elaboration Training (RET)

Schuell's Stimulation Approach

Sentence Production Program for Aphasia (SPPA)

Visual Action Therapy (VAT)

Anagram, Copy, and Recall Therapy (ACRT)

Background

ACRT, originally known as Anagram and Copy Treatment (ACT), trains the written modality as a compensatory strategy for communicating basic wants and needs (Beeson et al., 2002). The primary focus is the accurate spelling of single words for effective and functional communication. This therapy is suitable for aphasic patients who display limitations in both written and verbal output. Specifically, ACRT is appropriate for two groups of individuals: (a) those with poor verbal output who have severe aphasia and must rely on written expressions to communicate; and (b) those with good verbal output, who have mild aphasia with underlying spelling deficits. Such deficits may interfere with the activities of daily living, such as E-mailing, creating to-do lists, and taking telephone messages. For both groups of patients, individual words are trained. For the purposes of functional communication, it is recommended that the chosen words in ACRT be specific and relevant to the patient.

The authors used a cuing hierarchy that involved anagram letters and the act of copying single words repeatedly. It's based on "a cognitive model of single-word writing referred to as the lexical-semantic route" (Helm-Estabrooks & Albert, 2004), which is explained below.

The Process of Writing Single Words

1. First, a person perceives and recognizes the visual stimulus.

    For example, the image of a fish is shown. The following systems and tasks are then engaged.

2. Semantic System: Within a person's semantic system, there exists a conceptual representation of the word "fish." For example, *edible, fins, salt water, swims, gills.*

3. Graphemic Output Lexicon: People store the learned ability to spell in long-term storage, also known as the graphemic output lexicon.

4. Graphemic Output Buffer: The specific "spatially ordered lettered strings" (Helm-Estabrooks & Albert, 2004, p. 293) that accompany each learned word are stored in the graphemic output buffer, which is held in short-term memory.

5. Allographic Conversion: Learned spellings are converted to actual, physical letter forms.

6. Graphomotor Program: Finally, target words are physically written. "Fish." This is the last step to be activated (Helm-Estabrooks & Albert, 2004, p. 293).

Methodology

1. ACRT is best suited for patients with intact semantic, visual recognition, and graphomotor skills, but with remaining deficits in written naming skills. Graphomotor skills are defined as the process of converting graphemes to letters, and then writing those letters (Helm-Estabrooks & Albert, 2004).

2. The following pretests are given to determine appropriate candidates (Helm-Estabrooks & Albert (2004).

Test of Graphomotor Skills

Ask patient to copy the following sentence:

THE QUICK BROWN FOX JUMPS OVER THE LAZY DOG.

Test of Single-Word Reading Comprehension

Can the patient match a printed word to the visual representation of that word? The Boston Diagnostic Aphasia Examination (BDAE) (Goodglass & Kaplan, 1983) contains a reading subtest with a picture-word matching task. It is recommended that the patient scores with at least 75% accuracy.

Test of Written Confrontation Naming

Helm-Estabrooks and Albert (2004) suggest that specific pictures from the Boston Naming Test (BNT); (Kaplan, Goodglass, & Weintraub, 2000) be used to determine single-word spelling ability. These pictures are as follows:

1. Bed
2. Tree
3. Pencil
4. House
5. Comb
6. Saw
7. Broom
8. Camel
9. Bench
10. Dart
11. Canoe
12. Wreath
13. Igloo
14. Cactus
15. Pyramid

The clinician is instructed to present one picture at a time and have the patient write the name of the picture on an unlined 8½ × 11 piece of paper, using a black marker. The patient should demonstrate some understanding of the word form, that is, at least some letterforms should be present in the written production. For example, if a client is presented with the word "bench," and he or she is able to write "be" or "ben," this patient would be an appropriate candidate.

These 15 words also may be used post-treatment to demonstrate improvement. Therefore, these words should not be used in the course of treatment.

Test of Visual Memory

Helm-Estabrooks and Albert (2004) suggest the following two subtests:

1. The Visual Memory Span subtest of The Wechsler Memory Scale-3rd edition (Wechsler, 1997).
2. The Design Memory subtest of the Cognitive-Linguistic Quick Test (CLQT); (Helm-Estabrooks, 2001).

The patient should perform at or above the normal mean on the Visual Memory Span (WMS-III) subtest and normally on the Design Memory subtest of the CLQT (Helm-Estabrooks & Roberts, 2004).

Scoring Spelling Responses from the 15-Word List

Helm-Estabrooks & Albert (2004) developed a 0 to 5 scoring system. This ensures that if a patient partially spells a word right, he or she earns credit. This system is also appropriate for measuring change over the therapeutic course.

Note: some patients will make several attempts at the correct spelling of a word. Only count their final attempt when scoring. The scoring is unique to Helm-Estabrooks & Albert (2004).

0 = Totally incorrect, illegible, all letters wrong, substitution of a drawing

1 = Less than half correct or all right letters in the wrong order

2 = Half correct, or half letters in wrong order

3 = If more than half is correct, but not fully correct, or if two letters are reversed or letters are added to correct a word, score as:

4 = Self-corrected

5 = Fully correct on first attempt

Example: Possible scoring scenarios with the word "wreath:"

5 points = "wreath"

4 points = "wreth" then "wreath" (patient self-corrected)

3 points = "wraeth"

1 point = "wr"

0 points = "siss"

There are 15 total words from the BDAE, with the numerical score of "5" being the highest a patient can get. To determine the percentage correct, follow these steps:

15 (total words) × 5 (highest possible score) = 75 possible points

For example, if a patient earns a total of 46 points out of 75:

46/75 = .61 × 100 = 61% of possible points.

The following scoring criteria are from Helm-Estabrooks & Albert, 2004.

1. Do not penalize for a combination of uppercase and lowercase letters (e.g., bED).
2. For scoring spelling of words written:
   a. When the target word contains an odd number of letters, a partial score is either 3 or 1 but not a score of 2 (half correct).
      Example:
      "hos" for house = 3 points
      "hoh" for house = 1 point
   b. When a letter or two are added before or after the correct word, give 3 points.
      Example:
      "broomer" for broom = 3 points
   c. When the phonetic spelling is used, score as usual and describe the phonetic spelling.
      Example:
      "kom" for comb = 3 points (note use of phonetic spelling)
   d. When an acceptable semantic substitute is used, score it as a correct word.
      Example:
      "home" for house = 5 points
   e. Always score nonsense words as 0.
      Example:
      "meem" for igloo = 0 points

How to Prepare for an ACRT Session

It is advisable that a discussion be held with the patient's family to determine a priority list of words that will prove most beneficial to the patient. This may include objects, actions, or feelings relevant to the patient's life and ADL needs. Check with the family periodically to verify that these target words remain important, or if any new ones should be added to the list of treatment words.

ACRT follows a hierarchy, beginning with words that are short, regularly spelled and easily visualized. When these are mastered, the clinician may gradually add more complex and irregularly-spelled words. Once the target word list has been compiled and organized, these words may be pictorially represented through simple line drawings, personal photographs, and/or photographs clipped form magazines and newspapers.

Measuring Patient Response and Improvement with ACRT

The guidelines below will help the clinician determine if ACRT is effective for the patient:

1. ACRT is directly responsible for the patient's improvement in correctly spelling target words.
   a. A multiple baseline design may be used to determine if improvement is a direct result of ACRT. (Refer to Beeson, 1999; Beason et al., 2002; and Helm-Estabrooks & Albert, 2004) for more details.
2. "The effects of treatment are generalizing to the pre- and posttest BNT items" (Helm-Estabrooks & Albert, 2004, p. 299).
   a. Administer the 15 pictured items from the BNT to the patient after every 6 sessions of ACRT and at the end of treatment. Use the 0 to 5 scoring system.
3. The patient is improving their writing skills for functional communication purposes.
   a. Together with family members or caretakers, look at the patient's communication in the form of written notes, grocery lists, to-do lists, E-mails, and conversational exchanges.

References

Beeson, P. M. (1999). Treating acquired writing impairment: Strengthening grapheme representations. *Aphasiologoy*, *13*, 767–785.

Beeson, P. M., Hirsch, F. M., & Rewega, M. A. (2002). Successful single-word writing treatment: Experimental analyses of four cases. *Aphasiologoy*, *16*, 473–491.

Goodglass, H., & Kaplan, E. (1983). *Boston Diagnostic Aphasia Examination*. Hagerstown, MD: Lippincott Williams & Wilkins.

Helm-Estabrooks, N. (2001). *Cognitive Linguistic Quick Test*. San Antonio, TX: Psychological Corp.

Helm-Estabrooks, N., & Albert, M. (2004). *Manual of aphasia and aphasia therapy* (2nd ed.). Austin, TX: Pro-Ed (http://proedinc.com).

Kaplan, E., Goodglass, H., & Weintraub, S. (2000). *Boston Naming Test*. Philadelphia: Lea & Febiger.

Wechsler, D. (1997). *Wechsler Memory Scale–Third Edition*. San Antonio, TX: Psychological Corp.

Divergent Word Retrieval

Background

Divergent Word Retrieval is a cognitive stimulation approach. Divergent word retrieval (naming) requires that a person generate as many possible answers in relation to a given topic, such as a named category. For example, given the word "*farm*," how many different and appropriate farm animals can a person name? Or, given the topic "*fishing*," how many different words associated with this sport can a person name? As Davis (2000) noted, "In a divergent mode, we generate a quantity and variety of responses" (p. 87). Additionally, divergent naming tasks are open-ended (Chapey, 2001). Consequently, successful divergent naming involves the ability to generate many logical connections and cognitive flexibility (Guilford, 1967). For example, when provided the word *farm*, one must have the ability to change from very obvious associations with the word (animals, crops) to more indirect ones, e.g., *grain*, *bales*, etc. In a study by Grossman (1981), adults were asked to generate word lists for 10 categories, including furniture, tools, clothing, and sports. Adults without aphasia produced an average of 14.66 words for each category. Adults with fluent aphasia produced 6.71 words, while adults with nonfluent aphasia produced 5.29 words (Davis, 2000).

Rationale

Addressing this skill in the evaluation and treatment of patients with aphasia was indicated by Chapey, Ridgrodsky, and Morrison (1977). These researchers suggested that in addition to convergent tasks requiring one correct answer (such as with confrontation naming), divergent naming tasks were also needed to assess a "full range of word-finding conditions" (Davis, 2000, p. 87). Therefore, this task requires a patient to access memory in a broad sense of the term for stored semantic concepts, in order to offer a variety of appropriate or alternative responses (Chapey, Ridgrodsky, & Morrison (1977). Wepman (1972; 1976) supported the cognitive stimulation aspect to aphasia therapy. He believed that the use of discussions with a central topic and expanding on ideas within that topic should be focal points of aphasia treatment. It has been suggested that cognitive rehabilitation should go beyond the mere task of asking patients to recall a spoken word, which Lindfors (1987) describes as a lower-level cognitive process. Instead, the clinician should aim to stimulate higher-level cognitive processes. They should facilitate inferencing, thought organization, and problem-solving in the patient and that divergent thinking should one of the domains of cognition targeted for stimulation for the purpose of improving communication skills (Chapey, 1994).

Measurement

When assessing a patient's divergent naming skills, responses can be divided into two categories: (1) fluency (the number of responses a patient is able to generate); and (2) flexibility (the variety of the patient's responses) (Chapey, 1994). In some cases, it may be appropriate to look at the amount of unusual responses a patient is able to generate and the amount of important details a patient provides

about a relevant topic. Guilford (1967) refers to this as the creativity and the elaboration of the patient's responses on a naming task.

The "Chapey Speech and Language Checklist" (Chapey, 1994, pp. 113–114) presents the following tasks as possible to measure a patient's ability to produce divergent naming:

The patient is instructed to produce numerous logical possibilities/perspectives/ideas where appropriate.

1. List words beginning with a specified letter such as /s/ or /p/
2. Name objects within a group
3. List uses for a common object
4. List problems inherent in a common situation
5. Supply multiple possible solutions to problems
6. Suggest ways to improve a product
7. Specify details in planning an event, making a decision, or describing a procedure
8. Specify numerous episodes or substeps in a story
9. Elaborate

Chapey, Ridgrodsky, and Morrison (1977) and Chapey (1994) offer an example of how to score a patient's response when asked to name objects that can roll, with the patient's response as follows:

1. baseball
2. football
3. basketball
4. nickel
5. dime
6. quarter
7. car
8. truck

Fluency score = 8

Flexibility score = 3 (patient included 3 categories: balls, money, and transportation).

Additionally, if the above patient was to produce any words that were not relevant to the category of "objects that can roll," those words would not be counted.

The following list offers additional ideas for eliciting divergent naming (Chapey, 1994):

Common Situations: List problems that are inherent in a common situation.

Brick Uses: List many different uses for a common object.

Improve Product: Suggest ways to improve a particular object.

Consequences: List the effect of a new and unusual event.

Object Naming: List objects that belong to a broad class of objects.

Differences: Suggest ways in which two objects are different.

Similarities: Produce ways in which two objects are alike.

Word Fluency: List words that contain a specified word or letter.

Elaboration: List detailed steps needed to make a briefly outlined plan work.

References

Chapey, R. (1994). *Language intervention strategies in adult aphasia* (3rd ed.). Baltimore: Williams & Wilkins.

Chapey, R. (2001). *Language intervention strategies in aphasia and related neurogenic communication disorders* (4th ed.). Philadelphia: Lippincott, Williams & Wilkins.

Chapey, R., Rigrodsky, S., & Morrison, E. B. (1997). Aphasia: A divergent semantic interpretation. *Journal of Speech and Hearing Disorders, 42*, 287–295.

Davis, G. A. (2000). *Aphasiology: Disorders and clinical practice.* Needham Heights, MA: Allyn & Bacon (http://abacon.com).

Grossman, M. (1981). A bird is a bird is a bird: Making reference within and without superordinate categories. *Brain and Language, 12*, 313–331.

Guilford, J. P. (1967). *The nature of human intelligence.* New York: McGraw-Hill.

Lindfors, J.W. (1980; rev. 1987). *Children's language and learning.* Englewood Cliffs, NJ: Prentice-Hall.

Wepman, J. (1972). Aphasia therapy: A new look. *Journal of Speech and Hearing Disorders, 37*, 203–214.

Wepman, J. (1976). Aphasia: Language without thought or thought without language. *ASHA, 18*, 131–136.

High-Tech Alternative and Augmentative Communication (AAC) Devices

Background

The presence of word-finding deficits in patients with aphasia is well documented (Basso, 2003). Such difficulties have been shown to interfere with both daily living and social communication (Lesser & Algar, 1995). MossTalk Words® (MTW), developed at Moss Rehab (associated with the Albert Einstein Healthcare Network and Jefferson Health System of Pennsylvania), is a computer-based program that attempts to remediate word-finding deficits, by training comprehension and production of words at the word, phrase, and sentence levels.

Both MossTalk Words® and Lingraphica® are high-tech alternative and augmentative communication (AAC) devices. Such technology assumes that the concepts for functional communication remain unimpaired in patients, but there is a pronounced deficit in the ability to express such concepts (Helm-Estabrooks & Albert, 2004). With training, MTW and Lingraphica® provide patients with the ability to access a group of icons, pictures, and symbols that are compiled to represent words, phrases, and sentences. The patient first chooses specific icons and symbols and puts them together in logical order, in either phrase or sentence formats. As such, a patient is able to functionally communicate personal needs, wants, and interests.

Rationale

There are two fiscally-related problems that can occur over the course of First, the insurer sets limits on the duration of therapeutic intervention; and second, the patient's performance can sometimes plateau at a certain point in therapy, which does not present a sound case to the insurance companies for continued coverage (Fink, Brecher, Sobel, & Schwartz, 2005). As such, computer-based programs such as MTW and Lingraphica that seek to extend the course of rehabilitation to the home setting (once patient and caregivers are properly trained) seem like an appropriate solutions to the above noted problems. Another reason to use computer-based programs in the course of intervention is to supplement traditional therapy activities. Fink (2002) concluded that people with chronic aphasia who demonstrate significant phonologically based deficits can derive benefit from a computerized cued-naming methodology during treatment.

MossTalk Words® (MTW)

MTW is a software program that may be utilized in the clinic with the assistance of a speech-language pathologist or a trained volunteer, or it may be used independently in the patient's own home (Fink et al., 2005). MTW comes equipped with 340 vocabulary words and pictures, which may be presented in both the visual and auditory modalities.

Program Interfaces

There are three separate interfaces within the MTW program. They are as follows:

The "Standard Interface" contains three separate treatment modules. Each module contains an array of exercises which are organized in a hierarchy of easy-to-difficult tasks. For example, a more difficult task might include lower frequency vocabulary words or phonological foils that closely resemble the target production.

The "Customizing Interface" gives clinicians and caregivers the option of "preselecting" the items that will be included in the patient's exercise.

The "Assigned Exercises Interface" allows "patients to access preselected exercises independently" (Fink et al., 2005, p. 947).

Therapy Modules

(Adapted from Fink et al., 2005.)

Core-Vocabulary Module. Exercises include matching and naming tasks for the more severely impaired patient. This module contains a select group of vocabulary words associated with functional ADLs, such as common objects and the names of foods.

Multiple-Choice Matching Module. Includes exercises for strengthening vocabulary and comprehension in both speech and printed formats.

Cued-Naming Module. Single word production is the goal in this module. These exercises contain a cuing hierarchy and 8 possible cues (4 visual and 4 print), which may be used to facilitate word retrieval and production. The clinician assesses patient deficits and needs, and individualizes this module accordingly. The clinician can select the level of difficulty, the modality, the vocabulary and/or which cues to activate for a given exercise with a particular patient" (Fink et al., 2005, p. 946).

The cues are listed below (Ramsberger & Marie (2007).

Verbal cues:

1. first phoneme
2. sentence completion
3. definition
4. spoken word

Print cues:

1. first letter
2. written sentence completion
3. written definition
4. written word

Fink et al. (2005) instruct the clinician to carefully consider the type of chronic patient before selecting MTW. They advise that MTW is appropriate for patients primary progressive aphasia, and those who demonstrate semantically based deficits which are moderate in nature. This program is not suited for patients with a Wernicke's type aphasia, cognitive impairments, or patients who perseverate.

Both patients and clinicians alike gave high satisfactory remarks regarding MTW, highlighting ease of use and level of enjoyment. Initially, clinicians invested time to learn the software, but the general feeling was that this investment paid off long term, in that MTW saved clinicians time once the program was in use.

The use of computer technology is intimidating to some, especially those patients who are not regularly exposed to computers. Therefore, using a volunteer in the computer lab who is trained and/or supervised by a certified speech-language pathologist may provide an extra level of support that some patients require (Fink et al., 2005).

Lingraphica®

Lingraphica (www.lingraphica.com) was developed at the Boston VA Hospital nearly 30 years ago. Researchers first produced a program known as the Visual Communication System (VIC). Simple drawings that depicted categories of people, actions, and objects were produced on index cards. The patients then selected cards from these categories and laid them out to produce phrases and sentences as an alternative means of communication. In 1980, this system was adapted to the computer, and became known as Computer-Assisted Visual Communication (C-ViC) (Helm-Estabrooks & Albert, 2004; Shelton, Weinrich, McCall, & Cox, 1996; Steele, Kleczewska, Carlson, & Weinrich, 1992; Steele, Weinrich, Wertz, Kleczewska, & Carlson, 1989; Weinrich, Steele, Carlson, et al., 1989; Weinrich, Steele, Kleczewska, et al., 1989). This program was then adapted into what is known today as Lingraphica, a speech-generating device for use with patients with aphasia. Lingraphica was approved by Medicare in 2002. The cost of this device is reimbursed by most private insurance plans and many state Medicaid programs, including Medicare Part B, The Veterans Administration, Federal Supply Contract V797P-4886a, Aetna, the Department of Health and Human Services-USA.

Lingraphica® Program Features

Lingraphica® is a speech-generating computer software program that builds graphic symbols and pictures into phrases and sentences, which are then spoken aloud by a computer-generated and natural-sounding human voice. Essentially, the program integrates the visual and auditory modalities. It is flexible in that it provides multiple opportunities for extensive practice, and is appropriate for patients with varying levels of ability and who are at varying stages of recovery. The program is customizable in that it may be individualized to the patient based on his or her specific abilities, needs, and interests. Equipped

with a wide variety of vocabulary, patients may select specific words and build phrases and sentences to communicate basic wants and needs. Such phrases and sentences may then be saved and easily retrieved for later use. Lingraphica® also comes pre-equipped with standard phrases that may be used when eating in a restaurant or during doctors' visits.

Lingraphica® contains 240 different exercises at the easy, medium, and hard levels. It "offers unlimited speech practice, both at home and in therapy, through rehearsal and repetition of icons and phrases that use natural human voices" (www.Lingraphica.com). The program is to be administered by a trained and ASHA-certified speech-language pathologist.

The following information provides a review of methods for individualizing the program to the patient:

1. Small or large icons may be used, and this choice is based upon the patient's eyesight.
2. A patient may create their own icons.
   a. Example: Icons of grandchildren
      i. "My granddaughters Mary and Megan" would have two standard icons for "my" and "granddaughters," and two customized icons for "Mary" and "Megan."
   b. Two built-in cameras are included:
      i. Still camera: Patient may create still photos for personalized icons
      ii. Video camera: Patient may record video clips

Other features included in Lingraphica®:

1. Practice Videos
   a. Example: A patient may click on a video demonstration of production of the syllable "pa." When the patient clicks on this icon, a video reveals an up-close demonstration of a woman's lips producing "pa" two times. The idea is for the patient to then imitate this production.
   b. Other videos include additional practice phonemes and standard phrases.
2. Training Videos
   a. These are offered to the patients, to provide user-friendly video tutorials. The video depicts a person walking the patient step-by-step

through all program features, and this option is easily accessible through the "Help Menu.

3. Free Technical Support
   a. This is available toll-free, from 9 AM to 5 PM. A patient or caregiver may even email a question and will receive a response within 24 hours. The Web-site also offers downloadable manuals and reference guides. There is live internet support and even Web-based training over the Internet.

Lingraphica® is user friendly, with easy-to-understand drop-down menu items. A Spanish version is also included within the program for Spanish-speaking patients. Patients may even qualify for a free and no-obligation trial of Lingraphica®. To determine eligibility, the following steps are recommended.

1. The speech-language pathologist (SLP) working with the patient provides the patient's insurance information to Lingraphica® staff.
2. Lingraphica® staff runs a benefits check to make sure the device will be covered by the patient's personal insurance company.
3. Determination of eligibility is made within 24 hours.
4. If determined eligible, a loaner device is shipped out to the patient. (No paperwork is required).
5. The SLP receives over-the-phone training, which takes approximately one hour.
6. The trial typically takes 4 weeks to complete, with 2 devoted to the SLP providing the training, and 2 devoted to practice.

   During the four-week trial period, the patient is evaluated evaluated and introduced to the basic operations of the device by the SLP. Then the patient works independently with the device while also continuing therapy sessions. The patient and the clinician then decide if the device is appropriate for his/her communication needs (www.Lingraphica.com). This decision is aided by a built-in "Clinical Consultant" who also trains the SLP on the device.
7. If after the trial period it is determined that the program is appropriate, Lingraphica® will send a "Certificate of Medical Necessity" form to the patient and will simultaneously gather a physician-written prescription as well as insurance company authorization.
8. The loaner device is shipped back to Lingraphica®, free of charge.
9. After all the necessary paperwork has been processed, a customized Lingraphica® device is sent to the patient. This device will incorporate information specific to the patient, such as family member names, and individual needs and interests.
10. SLP's will receive 2.4 ASHA CEU's after completing the 4-week trial.

Evidence-Based Practice

"The Lingraphica has been proven effective in clinical studies, and is based on decades of aphasia research and technology development" (www.Lingraphica.com). This information has been documented in a number of publications and presentations, and can be obtained from the following link: http://www.lingraphica.com/slp/research.aspx

References

Basso, A. (2003). *Aphasia and its therapy.* New York: Oxford University Press.

Fink, R. B., Brecher, A., Schwartz, M. F., & Robey, R. R. (2002). A computer implemented protocol for treatment of naming disorders: Evaluation of clinician-guided and partially self-guided instruction. *Aphasiology, 16,* 1061–1086.

Fink, R. B., Brecher, A., Sobel, P., & Schwartz, M. F. (2005). Computer-assisted treatment of word retrieval deficits in aphasia. *Aphasiology, 19,* 943–954.

Helm-Estabrooks, N., & Albert, M. (2004). *Manual of aphasia and aphasia therapy* (2nd ed.). Austin, TX: Pro-Ed (http://proedinc.com).

Lesser, R., & Algar, L. (1995). Towards combing the cognitive neuropsychological and the pragmatic in aphasia therapy. *Neuropsychological Rehabilitation, 5,* 67–92.

Ramsberger, G., & Marie, B. (2007). Self-administered cued naming therapy: A single-participant investigation of a computer-based therapy program replicated in four cases. *American Journal of Speech-Language Pathology, 16,* 343–358.

Shelton, J. R., Weinrich, M., McCall, D., & Cox, D. M. (1996). Differentiating globally aphasic patients: Data from in-depth language assessments and production training using C-ViC. *Aphasiology, 10,* 319–342.

Steele, R. D., Kleczewska, M. K., Carlson, G. S., & Weinrich, M. (1992). Computers in the rehabilitation of chronic, severe aphasia: C-ViC 2.0 cross-modal studies. *Aphasiology, 6,* 185–194.

Steele, R. D., Weinrich, M., Wertz, R. T., Kleczewska, M. K., & Carlson, G. S. (1989). Computer-based visual communication in aphasia. *Neuropsychologia, 27,* 409–426.

Weinrich, M., Steele, R. D., Carlson, G. S., Kleczewska, M. K, Wertz, R. T., & Baker, E. (1989). Processing of visual syntax in a globally aphasic patient. *Brain and Language, 36,* 391–405.

Weinrich, M., Steele, R. D., Kleczewska, M. K, Carlson, G. S., Baker, E., & Wertz, R. T. (1989). Representation of "verbs" in a Computerized Visual Communication System. *Aphasiology, 3,* 501–512.

Lexical Retrieval and Sentence Production Programs

This section on lexical retrieval and sentence production presents seven interventional approaches designed to optimize lexical retrieval and sentence formulation in people with aphasia. The reader should be aware of the lack of efficacy studies that exist for most of the treatment approaches used with this patient population. However, for an extensive review of the evidence in lexical retrieval and sentence formulation approaches, we refer the reader to Aphasia: Treatment for Lexical and Sentence Production Skills (ASHA, 2004), an ASHA publication in collaboration with Special Interest Division 2, Neurophysiology and Neurogenic Speech and Language Disorders. The programs represented in this section are those that are most commonly used by clinicians and are reviewed in the above-mentioned ASHA publication.

Background

The therapeutic programs for lexical retrieval and sentence formulation all have common features as well as a common goal. Although the methodology varies, the functional outcome remains the same: to improve functional communication by optimizing the patient's access to the lexicon and then producing the most syntactically correct utterance allowable within the context of the severity of that patient's aphasia. Table E–1 summarizes the seven approaches. Each program is discussed in more detail to supplement the table.

Cuing Hierarchies

Linebaugh et al. (1983) stated that there are three basic principles of cueing hierarchies:

- Cues that elicit a response from the patient with the least amount of help from the clinician are the most desirable. They are the least powerful in the hierarchy.
- Cues should become less powerful as therapy continues.
- The patient must be trained to use self-cueing or "internal facilitators."

All cueing hierarchies must be client-specific. The ultimate goal is that the patient will require less powerful cues and will have learned to use that cue in response to other stimulus categories. For example, the client will self-cue with the first sound of a word across all semantic categories, not just the category used to train the technique in therapy. The clinician can use semantic cueing to facilitate the client's word retrieval, for example, by providing a descriptive cue for a word, or a sentence completion cue. Those cues are less powerful than having the client imitate the desired word. Therefore, they are higher up in the cueing hierarchy. One can also provide phonological cues, starting with the least powerful cue—providing a target word and phonological foils —proceeding to the most powerful cue, imitation. In between the two, one can cue the patient using a non-real rhyming word, or an articulatory cue. Linebaugh and Lehrer (1977) presented a modified cueing hierarchy by mixing types of cues. For example, they suggested giving the client the written representation of the first letter of the work along with an articulatory cue for the first phoneme. He also added gestural prompting to the hierarchy.

Table E–1. Selected Lexical Retrieval and Sentence Formulation Program Features

Author(s)	Program	Domain(s)	Primary Feature(s)
Patterson (2004)	Cuing Hierarchies	Semantic	The clinician uses cuing hierarchies in the semantic and/or phonological domains; gesture and grapheme-to-phoneme conversion can also be utilized
Raymer & Rothi (2001)	Comprehension Tasks That Facilitate Oral Naming	Semantic and Phonological	Naming tasks are constructed to tap into sound and meaning processes.
Boyle & Coehlo (1995)	Semantic Feature Analysis	Semantic	Improves lexical retrieval by facilitating access to semantic networks.
Garrett (1988)	Normal Sentence Production	Syntactic	Message Level, Functional Level, and Positional Level of Representation used to interpret sentential errors.
Schwartz et al. (1994)	Mapping Treatment	Semantic and Syntactic	This approach focuses on sentence construction and the link between meaning and structure.
Thompson (2001)	Treatment of Underlying Forms (TUF)	Syntactic	This approach was designed to improve sentence production by using noncanonical sentences.
Helm-Estabrooks & Albert (2004)	Melodic Intonation Therapy (MIT)	Prosodic	MIT uses melodic line, rhythm, and points of stress to facilitate sentence production.

Comprehension Tasks That Facilitate Oral Naming

Comprehension approaches to optimize word retrieval require the patient to perform tasks that facilitate the lexical processing function. For example, a patient may be asked about the meaning of a word; or asked to make a judgment about the sound characteristics of a target word. Other tasks include matching words to pictures, matching pictures to written words, and matching pictures to definitions. In all of these tasks, the receptive modality is used as a vehicle to facilitate word retrieval.

Semantic Feature Analysis

The underlying premise of Semantic Feature Analysis (Boyle & Coelho, 1995) is that by accessing the semantic network of a target word, the patient will be more likely to retrieve it since all like concepts are linked. The closer the concepts are, the stronger the

link. Therefore, patients are encouraged to produce words that are semantically related to the target word. Strongly associated words activate phonological information and the likelihood of target word production increases. One of the techniques used in the approach is the semantic feature diagram (Figure E–1).

Another important aspect of this approach is that the patient must produce all of the semantic features of the target work, even if it is named successfully. The intent is to strengthen the semantic network associated with that word.

Normal Sentence Production

Despite years of research efforts focused on producing a complete understanding of normal sentence production, that prize has been elusive. More current approaches to understanding the sentence production of aphasic speakers has led to a reconceptualization of not only that process but even the way that process is studied. For many years, the goal

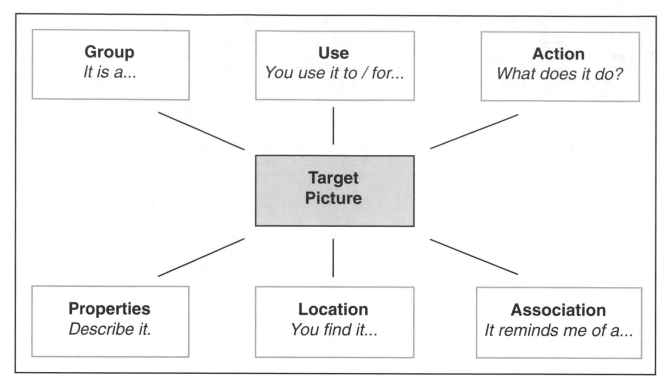

Figure E–1. Semantic feature analysis.

of studying sentence production in aphasia was to correlate the findings with anatomic data, so that speakers could be classified according to type, for example, Broca's, Wernicke's, and so forth. However, since the mid-1980s, researchers focused their energy on determining how normal sentence production was disrupted due to aphasia and left the classification issue behind. Borrowing from cognitive neuropsychology, language researchers found that cognitive analyses gave them a method to *interpret* aphasic language rather than *diagnosing* it.

Garrett (1988) developed a model of sentence production out of this context. He proposed three levels of cognitive representation used during sentence production: the *Message Level Representation*, the *Functional Level Representation*, and the *Positional Level Representation*. The Message Level is the level of meaning and intent. It is prelinguistic and the highest level of sentence production. It is at this level that the speaker decides to "say something." Consequently, speakers with difficulty at this level are unable to generate neither intent nor mean-

ing rendering them not functionally communicative. Speakers with difficulty at the Functional Level are able to produce grammatical morphemes, but have an impaired ability to express thematic roles, for example, *who is doing what to whom*. This level specifies word meanings for the content of the sentence, and multiple words are considered as candidates for selection. It also is argued that this level may be implicated in the noun/verb relationship. Thus, the choices made at this level will place some restrictions on the structure of the sentence, although at this level, the sentence contains no formal structure. Finally, there is the Positional Level. It is at this level that the syntactic phrase constituents impose structure on the forming sentence. Phonologically specified words are chosen, and free and bound morphemes are inserted. Impairment at this level produces a person with agrammatic verbal output.

Based on the above description of sentence production, a clinician would view the sentences produced by the aphasic speaker within that context and their errors also would be viewed from that perspective. The patient's therapy program would be constructed around and within the level error patterns were found. For example, a patient whose errors were noted to be at the Functional Level would be given tasks to facilitate thematic role production. The clinician would show the patient a picture of a scene, and ask the patient, *"Who is doing what to whom?"* A patient with difficulty at the Positional Level, would be engaged in tasks that focused on argument structure. The fewer arguments, the easier it is to generate a sentence.

Mapping Treatment

Mapping treatment aims to improve the link between meaning and structure at the sentence level. The underlying premise of this therapeutic approach is that the patient has lost the ability to convey meaning using noun-verb relationships, again indicating a problem with thematic roles. Therapy is focused on sentence production using probing questions: What is the verb? Who is doing the *verb-ing*? Who or what is the *verb-ing*? This Sentence Query Approach

becomes more specific over a three-month period. The patient is asked to:

1. Identify the verb
2. Identify the agent or actor by using a "who" query before the verb
3. Identify the patient/theme role by using "what" query after the verb
4. Identify the locative by using the "where" query
5. Ask questions about "when," "why," and "how"

Different sentence types are targeted ranging from simple subject + object NPs (*Susan drinks the soda*) to complex subject + object NPs (*The girl from the office was helping Mary's daughter*) (Figure E–2).

Treatment of Underlying Forms (TUF)

This therapeutic approach was developed to treat people with poor sentence comprehension and production, that is, agrammatism commonly associated with the non-fluent, Broca's type aphasia. Individuals

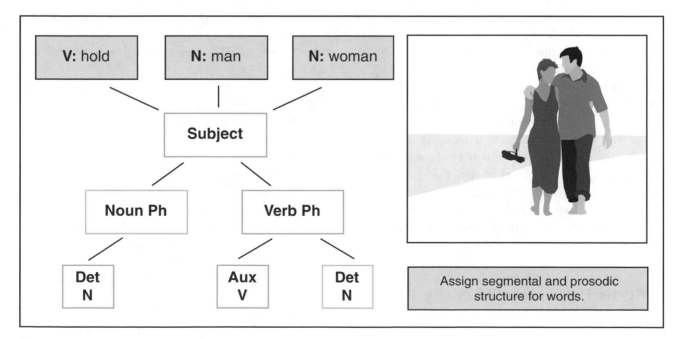

Figure E–2. An example of mapping treatment.

with agrammatism have a degraded grammatical structure, based on the type of sentences that they produce. They produce short S-V-O sentences with misordered or absent verb forms. They also have difficulty comprehending and producing *noncanonical* sentences, that is, sentences in which the NPs have been moved out of their *canonical* order, as they are in passives. Treatment of Underlying Forms (TUF) is a linguistic approach that focuses on training complex, non canonical sentences. The training hierarchy proceeds from complex to simpler sentence structures. The example below illustrates how the clinician facilitates simpler sentence construction from a more complex form. The stimulus is the sentence *It was the artist who the thief chased.*

1. Present cards (read aloud and repeat)
   [the thief] [chased] [the artist] [it was] [who]
2. Point to the verb, "This is <u>chase</u>, it is the action." Point to the theme, "This is the <u>thief</u>, the person doing the chasing." "This is the <u>artist</u>: the artist is the person who is chased."
3. The <u>who</u> card is placed next to the Theme card (the artist). Say, "To make a sentence, <u>who</u> is added next to the artist because the artist is the person who was chased."
   [the thief] [chased] [the artist] [who]
4. The theme (<u>the artist</u>) and the <u>who</u> cards are moved to the sentence initial position. "To make the correct sentence, these words are moved to the beginning of the sentence."
   [the artist] [who] [the thief] [chased]
5. The <u>it was</u> card is added to the beginning of the sentence. The examiner states: "<u>It was</u> is added to the sentence because it was the artist who the thief chased." The client reads and repeats:
   [it was] [the artist] [who] [the thief] [chased]
6. Sentence parts are rearranged in active sentence form together with the <u>it was</u> and <u>who</u> cards and the steps are repeated with the cards moving to form the target sentence.

Melodic Intonation Therapy (MIT)

In 1994, the Therapeutics and Technology Assessment Subcommittee of the American Academy of Neurology identified MIT as an "effective" treatment approach to language therapy. Melodic Intonation Therapy uses rhythmic intonations of phrases and sentences as the tool of language rehabilitation. The program is fully described in Helm-Estabrooks and Albert (2004).

The right hemisphere mediates musical stimuli and intonation (Shapiro, Grossman, & Gardner, 1981). It is speculated that the intact right hemisphere may have the ability to improve the language functions of the left hemisphere, which has been damaged, by utilizing the metrical functions of the right cortex. The underlying premise of MIT is that the right hemisphere is accessed to improve the fine motor movements for speech by using phrases that are intoned and paced syllable-by-syllable. The intoned model provided by the therapist is based on a melodic pattern, rhythm, and points of stress. Fluent phrases then become more possible when spoken with an exaggerated intonation than they would be without this approach.

It is best used with nonfluent aphasics who have poorly articulated output, and moderately preserved auditory comprehension. They also must have good motivation and attention span and be emotionally stable. Patients who respond well to this approach have an intact right hemisphere, with a unilateral left hemispheric stroke. Interestingly, patients who have poor repetition skills even for single words also respond well to MIT. There are three levels to MIT: Elementary, Intermediate, and Advanced.

- MIT Steps
  - Hand tapping with all intoned utterances
  - Clinician and patient intone and tap target phrase in unison
  - Clinician begins to fade participation at phrase midpoint
  - Clinician presents intoned utterance without allowing unison participation by patient
  - Patient signaled to repeat the intonation
- Elementary Level
  - Phrase is intoned but patient does not tap as he responds with target sentence to a question
- Intermediate Level

- A delay is introduced between the stimulus and response
- Advanced Level
  - Approximates normal speech intonation using "sprechgesang" or speech song.

References

ASHA Special Interest Division on Neurophysiology and Neurogenic Speech and Language Disorders. (2004). *Aphasia: Treatment for lexical and sentence production skills.* Rockville, MD: ASHA.

Boyle, M., & Coelho, C. A. (1995). Application of semantic feature analysis as a treatment for aphasic dysnomia. *American Journal of Speech-Language Pathology, 4,* 94–98.

Garrett, M. F. (1988). Processes in language production. In F. J. Newmeyer (Ed.), *Lingusitics: The Cambridge Survey: 111. Language: Psychological and biological aspects.* Cambridge: Cambridge University Press.

Helm-Estabrooks, N., & Albert, M. (2004). *Manual of aphasia therapy* (2nd ed.). Austin, TX: Pro-Ed.

Linebaugh, C., & Lehner, L. (1977). Cuing hierarchies and word retrieval: A treatment program. In R. H. Brookshire (Ed.), *Clinical aphasiology: Conferences proceedings.* Minneapolis, MN: BRK.

Linebaugh, C. W., Pryor, A. P., & Margulies, C. P. (1983). A comparison of picture descriptions by family members of aphasic patients to aphasic and nonaphasic listeners. In R. H. Brookshire (Ed.), *Clinical aphasiology conference proceedings.* Minneapolis, MN: BRK.

Patterson, J. P. (2001). The effectiveness of cueing hierarchies as a treatment for word retrieval impairment. *ASHA Special Interest Division 2 Newsletter, 11*(2), 11–18.

Raymer, A. H., & Rothi, L. G. (2008). Impairments of word comprehension and production. In R. Chapey (Ed.), *Language intervention strategies in aphasia and related neurogenic communication disorders* (5th ed.). Philadelphia: Wolters Kluwer.

Schwartz, M. F., Saffran, E. M., Fink, R. B., Meyers, J. L., & Martin, N. (1994). Mapping therapy: A treatment program for agrammatism. *Aphasiology, 8,* 9–54.

Shapiro, B., Grossman, M., & Gardner, H. (1981). Selective musical processing deficits in brain damaged populations. *Neuropsychologia, 19,* 161–169.

Thompson, C. K. (2001). Treatment of underlying forms: A linguistic specific approach for sentence production deficits in agrammatic aphasia. In R. Chapey (Ed.), *Language intervention strategies in aphasia and related neurogenic communication disorders* (4th ed., pp. 605–628).Philadelphia: Lippincott Williams & Wilkins.

See later section for more information on Melodic Intonation Therapy (MIT).

Life Participation Approach to Aphasia (LPAA)

Background

The long-term goal for any patient being treated using the LPAA approach is to reduce the barriers to the patient's participation in daily life activities and social relationships. In this approach, patients assume an active role in recovery. Patient participation occurs along a continuum that is ever changing, and reflects status at the time of treatment. This continuum evolves by first addressing immediate goals, such as asking nursing staff to use the bathroom, and later progresses to long-term goals, such as returning to a previous place of employment. LPAA targets any activities in the individual's daily life that are affected by aphasia, even if these activities do not involve communication.

LPAA is based on functional and pragmatic therapy approaches for patients with aphasia. Though it's important for a patients to regain the ability to communicate a need, LPAA goes a step further in that "the ultimate goal for intervention is reengagement into everyday society" (Chapey et al., 2000, p. 237). Although some aphasia therapies address life enhancement only after language deficits have been remedied, this approach identifies this goal from the beginning of treatment (Chapey, Duchan, Elman, Garcia, Kagan, Lyon, & Simmons-Mackie, 2008).

Methodology

The primary focus of this treatment approach is reengagement in life from the moment therapy begins. The patient is heavily involved in helping design a treatment plan that encompasses his or her goals of participation in daily life, thus creating a sense of empowerment. Two components are essential for re-engagement in daily life activities: a support system (family and friends) and patient motivation.

Five core values are central to LPAA, and should be integrated into assessment and intervention (Chapey et al., 2000). They are as follows:

1. Enhancement of life participation
   Together, the patient and clinician consider the following:
   a. To what extent can the patient with aphasia achieve life participation goals?
   b. To what extent does the aphasia interfere with achieving these goals?
   The clinician and patient work to improve short-term and long-term participation in life.
2. All those affected by aphasia are entitled to service. Aphasia affects more than just the patient; it also affects family members, colleagues, and friends. Therefore, LPAA aims to support those in close association, which may potentially facilitate improved quality of life for the patient. Examples of supportive services include:
   a. Training others how to support and facilitate communication (e.g., Kagan & Gailey, 1993; Lyon et al., 1997)
   b. Counseling regarding communication, life participation, and how to live life to the fullest with aphasia (e.g., Holland, 1999; Ireland & Wootten, 1996)
   c. Couples therapy—work on communication and relationship together (e.g., Boles, 1998)
   d. Group training in supported communication (e.g., training work colleagues, training health care practitioners) (Elman, 2000)
3. The measures of success include documented life enhancement changes. Outcome measures are a requirement of this treatment. The clinician is to assess:
   a. quality of life
   b. degree to which life participation goals have been met
4. Personal and environmental factors are targets of intervention. For those with aphasia, daily life can be disrupted in two areas:
   a. personal, or internal (includes physical, emotional, and psychological changes related to aphasia)
   b. environmental, or external (includes social and physical structures that impede ability to function in every day life activities)
   To determine target goals, these two areas must be continuously prioritized and assessed throughout therapy.
5. Emphasis is on availability of services as needed throughout all stages of aphasia therapy. Services are available from the onset, and end only when the patient and clinician agree that life participation goals have been met is formal treatment ended.

References

Boles, L. (1998). Conducting conversation: A case study using the spouse in aphasia treatment. ASHA SID 2 Newsletter. *Neurophysiology and Neurogenic Speech and Language Disorders*, pp. 24–31.

Chapey, R., Duchan, J. F., Elman, R. J., Garcia, L. J., Kagan, A., Lyon, J. G., et al. (2008). Life-participation approach to aphasia: A statement of values for the future. In R. Chapey (Ed.), *Language intervention strategies in aphasia and related neurogenic communication disorders* (5th ed.). Philadelphia: Wolters Kluwer/Lippincott Williams & Wilkins.

Elman, R. J. (2000). *Language disorders in adults grand rounds: Life participation approaches to aphasia*. Presented to the American Speech-Language-Hearing Association Convention, November, 2000.

Holland, A. (1999). Counseling adults with neurogenic communication disorders. [Videotape]. *ASHA* (Producer) Rockville, MD: American Speech-Language-Hearing Association.

Ireland, C., & Wootten, G. (1996). Time to talk: Counseling for people with dysphasia. *Disability and Rehabilitation, 18*(11), 585–591.

Kagan, A., & Gailey, G. (1993). Functional is not enough: Training conversation partners in aphasia. In A. Holland & M. Forbes (Eds.), *Aphasia treatment: World perspectives* (pp. 199–226). San Diego, CA: Singular.

Lyon, J. G., Cariski, D., Keisler, L., Rosenbek, J., Levine, R., Kumpula, J., et al. (1997). Communication partners: enhancing participation in life and communication for adults with aphasia in natural settings. *Aphasiology, 11*(7), 693–708.

Project Group. (2000). Life participation approach to aphasia: A statement of values for the future. *ASHA Leader, 5*, 4–6 (www.asha.org/publications/asha links.htm).

Melodic Intonation Therapy (MIT)

Background

Goldstein (1942) found that patients with severe aphasia were able to correctly speak words through the activity of singing. Clinicians then searched for therapy options which used melody and rhythm to stimulate speech production. Melodic Intonation Therapy (MIT) became the designated name for a therapy that capitalized on an intact right hemisphere and its role in processing intonation patterns.

Methodology

MIT follows a hierarchy of 3 levels, using the following target stimuli:

1. Multisyllabic words
2. Short, high-probability phrases
3. Increasing phonologically complex sentences

The first 2 levels are musically intoned. The third level is first intoned, then given exaggerated speech prosody, and, finally, spoken with normal speech prosody.

Preparation

1. Consider the communication needs of the patient and the family.
2. Pre-select stimulus items with associated pictures. Stimulus items should be high-probability syllables, phrases, or sentences. The *Sentence Production Program for Aphasia (SPPA)* provides appropriate hierarchies of syntactic difficulty.
3. Include MIT score sheet.
4. Sit across from the patient using a tabletop surface.
5. Begin with imperative sentences and sounds that are most visible, such as bilabials.
6. Rotate a wide variety of words, phrases, and sentences.

Presentation

1. Intone target stimulus slowly.
2. Use continuous voicing.
3. Include high and low tones associated with normal speech prosody (pitch).
4. Incorporate the rhythm and stress patterns found in normal speech.
5. Face patient so they may have visual access to your mouth.
6. Use right hand to hold the patient's left hand, tapping it on the table for each syllable.
7. Use left hand to signal to the patient when to listen and when to intone.
8. Progress consecutively through all steps of each level; no step may be skipped.
9. Allow 4 attempts of each step.

Scoring

For specific scoring procedures, refer to *Manual of Aphasia and Aphasia Therapy*, (Albert & Helm-Estabrooks, 2004). Essentially, a patient's score will determine progression to a more advanced level, discontinuation of therapy, or a complete discharge. Progression from one level to the next is dependent on the patient achieving a score of 90% or higher, using an assortment of target stimuli, during 5 consecutive therapy sessions.

Level 1. Pictures and environmental cues associated with the target stimuli are incorporated throughout. Hand tapping is used for all target stimuli productions.

1. Humming—The melody pattern of the stimulus item is hummed while a picture or environmental cue is provided. The patient's hand is tapped accordingly. Proceed to sing the stimulus item twice. No patient response is required.
2. Unison intoning—Intone stimulus item in unison. Hand tapping continues. If patient is unsuccessful after 4 repetitions, return to Step 1 and introduce a new stimulus item.
3. Unison intoning with fading—Begin in unison, intoning and hand tapping. Halfway through stimulus item, fade voice. The patient must complete the rest of the stimulus item independently.

4. Immediate repetition—Target stimulus is intoned and tapped as the patient listens. The patient independently repeats the target stimulus while hand tapping continues.

5. Response to probe question—Without hand tapping, quickly intone a probe question. For example, "What did you say?" The patient must then respond. Hand tapping may be provided only as the patient answers the question.

After all 5 steps are completed in succession, proceed back to Step 1 and introduce a new stimulus item.

Level 2. Delays between the target stimulus and the required response are introduced at this level. Pictures and environmental cues associated with the target stimuli, as well as hand tapping, are included. If patient is unable to complete a step with a delay, they are allowed to back up to a previous step. This will affect their overall score. If they are unsuccessful even with this, the clinician introduces a new target stimulus.

1. Introduction of target phrase—Using hand tapping, target phrase is intoned and repeated twice. No response is required.

2. Unison with fading—Begin in unison; tone and tap. Halfway through target phrase, fade voice as patient continues independently. Repeat target phrase twice in this format, even if the patient is successful.

3. Delayed repetition—Intone target phrase and tap. Provide a 6-second delay. Request repetition and hand tap as patient repeats, but do not provide verbal assistance. If patient fails, back up to Step 2: "Unison with fading." If this proves successful, attempt Step 3 again. If patient still fails, return to Step 1 and introduce new stimulus item.
   It is important to include a 6-second delay in between Steps 3 and 4.

4. Response to probe question—Without hand tapping, quickly intone a probe question.

For example, "What did you say?" The patient must then respond. Hand tapping may be provided simultaneously as patient answers the question. If patient is unsuccessful in providing a response,

back up to Step 3. If the patient proves successful at Step 3, wait 6 seconds before attempting the probe question once again. If the patient fails to answer this time, return to Step 1 and introduce a new stimulus item.

Level 3. This stage involves more complex utterances, with the aim to introduce normal prosody back into the patient's speech. A transitional step known as *Sprechgesang* (speech song) is first introduced to achieve the return to normal prosody, and is thought to sound similar to choral reading. The rhythm and stress of the target stimuli are emphasized. The previous intoning of stimuli is now replaced by the rising and falling pitches found in normal speech. Backing up to previous steps is also allowed in Level 3, but will affect the patient's overall score.

1. Delayed repetition—Intone target phrase while hand tapping, and pause for 6 seconds. The patient repeats once. Provide hand tapping should the patient require it. If the patient fails, back up one level to Step 2 "Unison with fading." If successful, attempt "Delayed repetition" in Level 3 again. If they fail, introduce new stimulus item.

2. Introducing "Sprechgesang"—Introduce target phrase twice. Do not sing; instead, exaggerate the rhythm and stress, doing so in a slow manner. Incorporate hand tapping. No response is required.

3. "Sprechgesang" (with fading)—Using sprechgesang, begin target phrase in unison with patient. Fade voice while patient completes phrase independently. If patient fails, repeat utterance in unison, but do not fade voice. Successful performance of this results in attempting Step 3 again. If patient fails after backing up, return to Step 1 with a new stimulus item.

4. Delayed spoken repetition—Target phrase is spoken to patient using normal prosody, without hand tapping. Allow for a 6-second delay. Patient must repeat with normal prosody. If successful, move to Step 5 after a 6-second delay. If patient is unsuccessful, attempt Step 4 again. If they continue to be unsuccessful, return to Step 1 and present new stimulus item.

Important: include a 6-second delay in between Step 4 and 5.

5. Response to a probe question—Ask a question using normal prosody. Patient should respond, also using normal prosody. If the patient fails, back up to Step 4 and then attempt Step 5 again. If they succeed, return to Step 1 and introduce a new stimulus item.

Measuring Response to MIT

The functional goal of MIT is to improve the communication skills of patients with significant expressive impairment. Progress can be measured by using a variety of tools, including: giving a close family member the Communication Questionnaire (Helm-Estabrooks, 1996) before and after MIT; standardized aphasia tests which require narrative descriptions of pictures, such as the "Cookie Theft" in the Boston Diagnostic Aphasia Examination (BDAE); and pre- and post-MIT speech samples of the patient.

Narrative Story Cards

Background

The process of telling and re-telling a story involves the interaction of cognitive and linguistic skills. This process includes word-retrieval, correct word morphology, appropriate sentence syntax, narrative cohesion, working memory, pragmatic awareness, and visual perception. Narrative Story Cards as an approach is appropriate for adolescent and adult populations who have brain damage and who may experience deficits in narrative discourse.

Methodology

The Narrative Story Cards include 15 separate stories to facilitate planning, organization, word-retrieval, syntax, topic maintenance, and working memory. The stories contain emotional content, which is thought to stimulate memory function. Included in each set are pictures, a text, and titles.

The Narrative Story Cards Range in Order of Complexity from 3 to 5 Cards Each

6 story sets include 3 cards each

4 story sets include 4 cards each

5 story sets include 5 cards each

All sets include a story sheet to be used along with the cards for telling and re-telling the story. A content unit checklist associated with each story is also included. This is used to record client responses and to determine narrative discourse skills (Helm-Estabrooks & Nichols, 2002). For example, in the story *"Casino Luck,"* card 3 reads: "It's now four o'clock and Joe has just a few pennies left. Three hours and no luck!"

The following information units are included on the checklist.

1. four
2. o'clock
3. Joe/he
4. has
5. few
6. pennies
7. three
8. hours
9. no luck

If the client mentions any of the above words, a check mark is placed in the column to the right. The final score is calculated by adding the patient's total information units and dividing this number by the total number of possible units. If the total number of possible units was 55, but the patient only expressed 23 units, the final score would be 23/55 or 42%.

List of Tasks

The following list of tasks are suggested for use with Narrative Story Cards (Helm-Estabrooks & Nicholas, 2002).

1. Sequencing the cards
2. Telling story once given the cards

3. Retelling the story and making up a new ending
4. Giving the story a title
5. Comprehension for titles read
6. Comprehension of story read, matched to correct pictures
7. Writing story given information
8. Writing story without word prompts
9. Retelling story in written form
10. Auditory comprehension of information

References

Helm-Estabrooks, N., & Albert, M. (2004). *Manual of aphasia and aphasia therapy* (2nd ed.). Austin, TX: Pro-Ed (http://proedinc.com).

Helm-Estabrooks, N., & Nicholas, M. (2002). *Narrative story cards*. Austin, TX: Pro-Ed.

Goldstein, K. (1942). *After effects of brain-injuries in war: Their evaluation and treatment.* New York: Grune & Stratton.

Nonsymbolic Movements for Activation of Intention (NMAI)

Background

The self-initiation of complex behaviors has its origins in the presupplementary motor area, an intentional mechanism center within the brain (Picard & Strick, 1996). Complex behaviors include language tasks such as word generation and hand gesturing, which individuals with nonfluent aphasia have difficulty initiating due to lesions in that area. After a stroke in the left hemisphere, language production mechanisms may move to the right hemisphere whereas the intention mechanisms remain in the left hemisphere. According to the theory, this may create a disconnection between the two communicating centers. It is this phenomenon that may explain the difficulty of word generation found in nonfluent aphasics.

Previous research has highlighted a successful intervention technique for aphasia, using American Indian Sign Language during verbal naming tasks (Hoodin & Thompson, 1983; Kearns, Simmon, & Sis-terhen, 1982; Pashek, 1997; Skelly, Schinsky, Smith, & Fust, 1974). This therapy required the patient to name objects while simultaneously performing a hand gesture with their nondominant hand. They found that naming accuracy improved using this technique. However, the authors of a more recent pilot study, suggested that the complex hand movements actually activated the intentional centers in the right hemisphere, and as a result, helped with word production (Richards, Singletary, Rothi, Koehler, & Crosson, 2002). If these complex hand movements activated intentional centers in the right hemisphere, maybe they could potentially activate the initiation of language. Essentially, switching initiation centers to the same side as the production centers (initiated by complex hand movement in the nondominant hand) would improve naming accuracy.

Treatment

The treatment protocol is described below (Richards et al., 2002).and it can be conducted could be in the therapy session with a few modifications. In lieu of the computer program, the clinician could provide his or her own black and white line drawings and accompanying words, as well as a stopwatch. The treatment seeks to stimulate right hemisphere initiation centers through the use of complex hand gestures in the nondominant hand. The phases are in succession, beginning with the patient receiving external cues to the patient receiving no cues and creating their own non-symbolic hand gesture.

Treatment in the research study consisted of three phases. Each phase included ten 45-minute sessions. During each session, the clinician presented and named a set of 50 black and white line drawings for a total of 150 pictures for all three phases. The 50 words in each phase were broken down into 15 high-frequency, 15 medium-frequency, and 20 low-frequency words. The clinician began each trial by clicking a mouse button, thereby activating a timer. When the black and white line drawing appeared on the computer monitor, the patient was to name the picture as quickly as possible. If the patient was unable to produce the correct name within 20 seconds, the computer program recorded an incorrect response and moved on to the next probe item.

Phase I of Intention Treatment (10 sessions)

The same set of 50 line drawings is trained each day of the treatment phase.

1. Patient sits at desk. Body and head face straight forward.
2. Computer monitor is positioned in front of patient.
3. Clinician activates program by clicking mouse.
4. Image of a star appears in center of computer screen along with a 1000-Hz tone.
5. Patient presses a button inside a box to his left to make the star and tone go away.
6. After a 2-second delay, a black and white drawing appears and the timer begins.
7. Correct naming of the object prompts the clinician to click the mouse, which ends the timer and removes the picture from the screen.
8. Incorrect naming of the object prompts the clinician to name a picture while making a circular gesture with the left hand.
9. Patient repeats this word and imitates the hand gesture.

Phase II of Intention Treatment (10 sessions)

A different set of 50 line drawings is introduced.

1. Patient seated in same position as in Phase I.
2. Clinician activates program by clicking mouse.
3. Star appears in the center of the screen, without tone.
4. Patient presses button inside a box to his left to make the image go away.
5. After a 2-second delay, the black and white drawing appears and the timer begins.
6. Incorrect responses are corrected in the same way as Phase I.

Phase III of Intention Treatment (10 sessions)

A different set of 50 line drawings is introduced.

1. Patient seated in same position as in Phase I.

2. Clinician activates program by clicking mouse.
3. Star appears in the center of the screen, without tone.
4. Patient is to produce a meaningless hand gesture with the left hand 3 times.
5. Clinician clicks mouse button to begin presentation of line drawings.
6. Incorrect responses are corrected in the same way as in Phases I and II.

Results

The authors of the study employed the single subject A-B design. Two tests were administered: the Rey-Osterrieth Complex Figure Test (Meyers & Meyers, 1995), and the Block Design Subtest of the Wechsler Adult Intelligence Scale-Revised Edition (WAIS-R) (Wechsler, 1981).

In one subject, gesturing with the left hand appeared to facilitate word generation, aiding in motor production and reducing the patient's groping for words. There was overall improvement in functional communication, as reported by his caretakers. Additionally, there was carryover of the hand gestures to everyday situations.

As there were only three participants in the study, the authors caution against generalizing the findings to the broader population. Additionally, they noted limitations associated with an A-B design. Although results of this study were promising, further investigation is needed.

References

Hoodin, R. B., & Thompson, C. K. (1983). Facilitation of verbal labeling in adult aphasia by gestural, verbal, or verbal plus gestural training. *Clinical Aphasiology*, *13*, 62–64.

Kearns, K., Simmon, N. N., & Sisterhen, C. (1982). Gestural Sign (Amer-Ind) as a facilitator of verbalization in patients with aphasia. *Clinical Aphasiology*, *12*, 183–191.

Meyers, J. E., & Meyers, K. R. (1995). *Rey complex figure test and recognition trial*. Lutz, FL: Psychological Assessment Resources.

Pashek, G. (1997). A case study of gesturally cued naming in aphasia: Dominant versus nondominant hand training. *Journal of Communication Disorders, 30*, 349–366.

Picard, N., & Strick, P. L. (1996). Motor areas of the medial wall: A review of their location and functional activation. *Cerebral Cortex, 6*, 342–353.

Richards, K., Singletary, F., Gonzalez Rothi, L. J., Koehler, S. (2002). Activation of intentional mechanisms through utilization of nonsymbolic movements in aphasia rehabilitation. *Journal of Rehabilitation Research and Development, 39*, 445–454.

Skelly, M., Schinsky, L., Smith, R., & Fust, R. S. (1974). American Indian (AmerInd) Sign as a facilitation of verbalization for the oral verbal apraxic. *Journal of Speech and Hearing Disorders, 39*, 445–456.

Wechsler, D. (1981). *The Wechsler Adult Intelligence Scale*. New York: The Psychological Corporation.

Promoting Aphasics' Communicative Effectiveness (PACE)

Background

PACE therapy (Davis, 2007; Wilcox & Davis, 1977) attempts to mimic the natural exchange of conversation between two people. As noted by Wertz (1984), PACE focuses on the *context* of language rather than *content*. In the program, both the clinician and patient assume equal responsibility in communication, much like conversational partners do everyday during conversation. Both communicators take turns sending and receiving messages. PACE does not require a specific modality of communication. Instead, the patient is free to communicate through whatever modality he or she chooses. As noted by Peach (2008), PACE falls within the category of Functional Communication Treatment (FCT) and has been used with globally aphasic patients. In this model, improving the patient's ability to communicate individual and daily needs is the central theme.

Methodology

PACE follows a hierarchy whereby complexity of communication and abstraction of the message increases as therapy continues. Picture cards are used as message-generating stimuli and include the following hierarchy:

1. Phase I uses everyday object picture cards
2. Phase II uses verb picture cards
3. Phase III uses story-sequence picture cards

The clinician is free to choose whatever images he or she wishes to use.

PACE is composed of the following principles of conversation.

1. *New information is exchanged between clinician and patient.*
   A stack of picture cards is placed face down between the patient and the clinician. One takes a turn describing the picture and the other deciphering the message. The positive part of both partners assuming equal roles in communication is that the clinician can model appropriate responses for the patient to imitate when it is their turn. Secondly, the clinician can model communication modalities that the patient may not be using, but is capable of using. Picture cards should follow the aforementioned hierarchy, beginning with everyday object picture cards, moving to verb picture cards, and finally, using story-sequence picture cards. An alternative method is to use a barrier screen between the clinician and patient (Muma, 1978). Through dialogue, each person should end up with identical "boards." For example, if the clinician and patient each have a piece of paper with identical objects, both people will communicate the appropriate information in order to end up with identical images or configurations. For more information on this method, refer to Newhoff and Apel (1990).

2. *Equal participation of patient and clinician.*
   Both people take turns sending and receiving messages. In this way, therapy resembles a natural conversation.

3. *The communication mode is chosen by the patient.*
   Instead of the clinician training a specific communication modality, the patient chooses their response mode. Drawings, speaking, writing, pantomiming, gesturing, and pointing at objects are all accepted modalities. Leaving options open permits greater chances of patient success.

4. *Functional feedback is provided.*
In the same way that a conversational partner would respond to their partner's message, a clinician responds to the patient. If the clinician successfully understood the patient's message, she or he will respond appropriately. This gets the clinician away from the traditional role of rating a patient's response as either correct or incorrect. If the patient has accurately conveyed the information, the clinician will understand it and give reinforcement in the form of a response.

References

Davis, G. A. (2007). *Aphasiology: Disorders and clinical practice* (2nd ed.). Boston: Allyn & Bacon.

Muma, J. R. (1978). *Language handbook: Concepts, assessment and intervention.* Englewood Cliffs, NJ: Prentice-Hall.

Newhoff, M., & Apel, K. (1990). Impairments in pragmatics. In L. L. Lapointe (Ed.), *Aphasia and related neurogenic language disorders* (pp. 221–233). New York: Thieme Medical.

Peach, R. K. (2008). Global aphasia: Identification and management. In R. Chapey (Ed.), *Language intervention strategies in aphasia and related neurogenic communication disorders* (5th ed.). Philadelphia: Wolters Kluwer/Lippincott Williams & Wilkins.

Wertz, R.T. (1984). Language disorders in adults: State of the clinical art. In A. Holland (Ed.), *Language disorders in adults*. San Diego, CA: College-Hill Press.

Wilcox, M. H. & Davis, G. (1977). Speech act analysis of aphasic communication in individual and group settings. In R. H. Brookshire (Ed.), *Clinical aphasiology conference proceedings* (pp. 166–174). Minneapolis, MN: BRK.

Response Elaboration Training (RET)

Background

Response Elaboration Training (RET) is a method that attempts to mimic natural communication and promote generalization of responses (Kearns, 1985, 1990). RET is different from traditional production methods in that no predetermined set of responses are trained. Instead, the clinician uses patient-initiated responses as the main substance of therapy. These responses are shaped and expanded by the clinician to increase the length and richness of patient utterances. The end goal is to increase a patient's ability to self-initiate responses and become an independent communicator. RET is based on a "loose training" method developed by Stokes and Baer (1977). Loose training procedures create a treatment environment that provides stimuli that are found in the natural environment, allows for response variations that occur in that environment, thus promoting generalization outside the therapy room (Marshall, 2008). The literature does show evidence of generalization with this treatment methodology (Kearns, 1985; Kearns & Potechin, 1988).

Methodology

Action picture cards are the stimuli used in RET, typically consisting of transitive and intransitive verbs. (The clinician may choose his or her own imagery under these guidelines.) Instead of providing a simple description of the action picture, patients should be encouraged to draw on their world knowledge and personal experience in formulating a response.

The clinician follows the steps below for elaborating a patient's self-initiated utterances, as outlined by Kearns (1990):

1. An initial response is elicited to a picture stimulus.
2. This response is modeled and reinforced by the clinician
3. "Wh" cues are provided to prompt clients to elaborate on their initial responses.
4. The subsequent client-attempted response is reinforced, and then sentences that combine initial and subsequent responses to a given stimulus picture are modeled.
5. A second model of sentences that combine previous responses are modeled and then the client is instructed to repeat the sentence.
6. Repetitions of combined sentences are reinforced, and a final sentence model is provided.

Example

Table E–2 provides an example of the clinician's and patient's role in RET. The picture stimuli provided to

Table E–2. RET Steps and Responses

RET Steps	Clinician's Stiimulus	Patient's Response	Clinician's Feedback
1. Elicit initial verbal response to picture.	Line drawing of simple event (man with a broom) "Tell me what's happening in this picture."	"Man . . . sweeping."	
2. Reinforce, model, and shape initial response.			"Great. The man is sweeping."
3. Wh-cue to elicit elaboration of initial response	"Why is he sweeping?"	"Wife . . . mad."	
4. Reinforce, model, and shape the two patient responses combined.			"Way to go! The man is sweeping the floor because his wife is mad."
5. Second model and request repetition.	"Try and say the whole thing after me. Say, 'The man is sweeping the floor because his wife is mad'."	"Man . . . sweeping . . . wife . . . mad."	"Good job."
6. After reinforcement, elicit a delayed imitation of the combined response.	"Now, try to say it one more time."	"The man . . . sweeping because his wife . . . mad."	

Sources: Kearns and Potechin Scher, 1988; Kearns and Yedor, 1991.

the patient in this example shows a man sweeping the floor.

References

Chapey, R. (1994). *Language intervention strategies in adult aphasia* (3rd ed.). Baltimore: Williams & Wilkins.

Kearns, K. P. (1985). Response elaboration training for patient initiated utterances. In R. H. Brookshire (Ed.), *clinical aphasiology conference proceedings* (pp. 196–204). Minneapolis, MN: BRK.

Kearns, K. P. (1990). Broca's aphasia. In L. L. Lapointe (Ed.), *Aphasia and related neurogenic language disorders.* New York: Thieme Medical.

Kearns, K. P., & Potechin, G. (1988). The generalization of response elaboration training effects. In T. Prescott (Ed.), *Clinical aphasiology* (pp. 223–246). Boston: College-Hill Press.

Kearns, K. P., & Yedor, K. (1991). An alternating treatments comparison of loose training and a convergent treat-

ment strategy. In T. E. Prescott (Ed.), *Clinical Aphasiology* (Vol. 20, pp. 223–238). Austin, TX: Pro-Ed.

Marshall, R. C. (2008). Early management of Wernicke's aphasia: A context-based approach. In R. Chapey (Ed.), *Language intervention strategies in aphasia and related neurogenic communication disorders* (5th ed.). Philadelphia: Wolters Kluwer/Lippincott Williams & Wilkins.

Stokes, T., & Baer, D. M. (1977). An implicit technology of generalization. *Journal of Applied Behavior Analysis, 10,* 349–367.

Schuell's Stimulation Approach

Background

After two decades of working with people with aphasia, Hildred Schuell developed the Stimulation-Facilitation Approach, also known as "Schuell's Stimulation Approach." She believed that language was neither lost nor destroyed in the patient with aphasia. Rather, she believed that language was no longer easily retrieved due to a damaged, less efficient system. Therefore, her therapy approach does not "reteach" language. Instead, the speech-language pathologist is to "stimulate adequate functioning of disrupted processes" (Schuell et al., 1955).

Coelho, Sinotte, and Duffy (2008) have written a chapter about Schuell's stimulation approach to rehabilitation. It is "an approach to the treatment of aphasia that places its primary emphasis on the stimulation presented to the patient" (p. 403). The goal is to help maximize the patient's reorganization of language.

According to research, a majority of patients with aphasia demonstrate weaknesses in the auditory modality (Duffy & Ulrich; 1976; Schuell et al., 1964; Smith, 1971). The stimulation approach encourages speech-language pathologists to strengthen language input and output. The intensive stimulation involved in this approach is thought to strengthen the disrupted neural pathways important to language processing.

Schuell did not classify aphasic patients into the orderly and traditional paradigms, such as expressive aphasia, receptive aphasia, and so forth. Instead, the aphasias were classified according to three other criteria: the severity of the language impairment, the presence sensory or motor deficits, and the patient's prognosis (Duffy & Coelho, 2001).

System of Classification

Schuell's system of categorizing aphasia included the following (Jenkins et al., 1975):

- Simple aphasia
- Aphasia with visual involvement
- Aphasia with persisting dysfluency
- Aphasia with scattered findings
- Aphasia with sensorimotor involvement
- Aphasia with intermittent auditory imperception
- Irreversible aphasia syndrome

The following general principles are important to remediation (Brookshire, 1992; Schuell, 1974; Schuell et al., 1964).

1. Use intensive auditory stimulation. Pair visual and auditory modalities together.
2. Stimulation should be sufficient enough to reach the brain.
3. Sensory stimulation should be repetitive.
4. Stimuli provided to the patient should evoke a response.
5. Try for a maximum number of responses from the patient.
6. Provide feedback to the patient about his or her progress.
7. Treatment should be systematic and often.
8. Each session should follow a hierarchy from easy to more difficult tasks.
9. The clinician should have a variety of materials on hand to help ward off boredom if using drill-style formats.

Where to Begin Therapy (Brookshire, 1992)

1. The clinician should begin at a level where the patient is demonstrating only minor deficiencies.
2. Begin with tasks in which the patient's responses are correct about 60 to 80% of the time.
3. Increase the level of difficulty when performance reaches 90%.

The use of standardized measures can measure baseline performance and pinpoint an appropriate starting point. For instance, if a patient is incorrect 50% of the time during a two-step direction task on a standardized test, make that a task for therapy.

Tasks Highlighting the Patient's Auditory Capabilities

1. Point-to tasks
2. Following directions of varied length and complexity
3. Answering yes/no questions and verify sentences
4. Response switching (rapidly changing directions to follow, questions to answer)

Tasks Highlighting the Patient's Verbal and Auditory Capabilities

1. Repetition tasks
2. Sentence or phrase completion

3. Verbal association
4. Answering wh-questions
5. Connected utterances in response to single words (define words and complete phrases)
6. Retelling paragraphs and stories
7. "Self-initiated" or conversational verbal tasks (name pictures, describe function of objects, describe activities, etc.)

Tasks Targeting the Patient's Reading and Writing Abilities

1. Reading (match written words and sentences to pictures, identify letters named, read in unison, fill in missing words in sentences, read aloud and retell, etc.).
2. Writing (copy forms, letters, words, write letters to dictation, write known information, fill in missing words in sentences, write down essential information told, etc.).

References

Brookshire, R. H. (1992). *An introduction to neurogenic communication disorders* (4th ed.). St. Louis, MO: Mosby Year Book.

Chapey, R. (1994). *Language intervention strategies in adult aphasia* (3rd ed.). Baltimore: Williams & Wilkins.

Coelho, C. A., Sinotte, M. P., & Duffy, J. R. (2008). Schuell's stimulation approach to rehabilitation. In R. Chapey (Ed.), *Language intervention strategies in aphasia and related neurogenic communication disorders* (5th ed.). Philadelphia: Wolters Kluwer/ Lippincott Williams & Wilkins.

Duffy, J. R., & Coelho, C. A. (2001). Schuell's stimulation approach to rehabilitation. In R. Chapey (Ed.), *Language intervention strategies in aphasia and related neurogenic communication disorders* (4th ed.). Philadelphia: Lippincott Williams & Wilkins.

Duffy, R. J., & Ulrich, S. R. (1976). A comparison of impairments in verbal comprehension, speech, reading, and writing in adult aphasics. *Journal of Speech and Hearing Disorders, 41*, 110–119.

Jenkins, J., Jimnez-Pabn, E., Shaw, R., & Sefer, J. (1975). *Schuell's aphasia in adults* (2nd ed.). New York: Harper & Row.

Schuell, H. (1974). The treatment of aphasia. In L. F. Sies (Ed.), *Aphasia theory and therapy: Selected lectures and papers of Hildred Schuell.* Baltimore: University Park Press.

Schuell, H., Carroll, V., & Street, B. S. (1955). Clinical treatment of aphasia. *Journal of Speech and Hearing Disorders, 20*, 43–53.

Schuell, H., Jenkins, J., & Jiménez-Pabón, E. (1964). *Aphasia in adults: Diagnosis, prognosis and treatment.* New York: Harper & Row.

Smith, A. (1971). Objective indices of severity of chronic aphasia in stroke patients. *Journal of Speech and Hearing Disorders, 36*, 167–207.

Sentence Production Program for Aphasia (SPPA)

Background

According to Helm-Estabrooks and Nicholas (2000), sentence-level deficits are a diagnostic indicator for nonfluent aphasia. In a previous study Gleason et al. (1975) using story-completion tasks with patients who displayed Broca's Aphasia and agrammatism, concluded that the patients were not lacking in *knowledge* of syntax; but *access* to that knowledge (Davis, 2000). This study was the inspiration behind training a hierarchy of syntactic structures in the SPPA program, beginning with easy-to-produce structures and ending with more complex ones. Results of the study indicted that patients had the ability to produce a wide variety of syntactically correct utterances (Helm-Estabrooks & Albert, 2004)

The overarching goal of SPPA is to improve functional communication skills in the patient's daily interactions, such as making requests, conversing socially with others, and asking questions. Potential candidates for SPPA include patients who are nonfluent with agrammatic speech patterns, and who have relatively spared auditory comprehension. SPPA seeks to reduce the impact of agrammatism on spoken communication by improving the patient's ability to speak in increasingly longer and more complex sentences.

Program Overview

SPPA contains eight sentence types that are presented in a hierarchy of increasing difficulty, with 15 target sentences each and two separate levels of difficulty. A spiral-bound booklet contains all materials needed for the SPPA program. This includes stories, pictures, and target stimuli. In addition to the published version (Helm-Estabrooks & Nicholas, 2000), clinicians may use their own target stimuli, pictures and stories, as long as they follow the sentence-type hierarchy.

Picture Stimuli

Pictorial representations include three different families of various ethnic backgrounds engaged in verbal interactions during everyday situations. For example, to functionally demonstrate what to do in an emergency, an illustration of a family is shown responding to an accident, reaching for the phone. The target phrase is, "Call 911."

Difficulty Levels

There are two difficulty levels for each picture. One provides a clinician model and the other one does not provide a model.

Level A: Clinician model provided

Patient repeats a modeled sentence in response to a question.

Level B: No clinician model provided

Patient completes the story with the target sentence, without requiring the use of a clinician model.

Example of Level A and Level B

Sentence Type 1: Imperative Intransitive

Sample Target Phrase: "Wake up."

Level A: Nick's school bus arrives in 15 minutes and Nick is still asleep, so his mother tells him, "Wake up!" What does his mother say?

Level B: Nick's school bus arrives in 15 minutes and he is still asleep. So what does his mother tell him to do?

Presentation Suggestions

a. Speak in a natural voice.
b. Use a slow, natural rhythm with appropriate pauses and intonation.
c. Level A probe: Pause right before saying the target stimuli so patient is attuned to it, therefore enhancing his or her ability to repeat it.
d. Level B probe: Use rising intonation at the end of reading so patient is clued in to when it's time to complete the story.
e. If patient fails to respond, one repetition only is granted at each level.
f. Upon successful response to Level A, immediately administer Level B to the patient.
g. Once an 85% accuracy level is achieved with Level B, present the 15 items for each sentence type using only Level B.
h. Progress to next sentence type in hierarchy.

The 8 Sentence Types

(Helm-Estabrooks & Albert, 2001.)

1.	Imperative intransitive	"Wake up."
2.	Imperative transitive	"Drink your milk."
3.	Wh-interrogative (what & who)	"What are you watching?"; "Who is coming?"
4.	Wh-interrogative (where & when)	"Where is the hospital?"; "When are we landing?"
5.	Declarative transitive	"I teach school."
6.	Declarative intransitive	"He swims."
7.	Comparative	"She's taller."
8.	Yes/No questions	"Is it sad?"

Scoring

Patients may receive a score of 0, .5, or 1. The manual includes specific instructions, as well as scoring sheets that may be reproduced. For more information, refer to Helm-Estabrooks and Albert (2004).

Measuring Progress

The functional goal of SPPA is to reduce the patient's agrammatism and to improve ability to communicate using more syntactically complex sentences. To assess progress, formal measures such as the Communicative Effectiveness Profile (CEP) (Menn, Ramsberger, & Helm-Estabrooks, 1994) may be used. It also is important to obtain feedback from caregivers who interact with the patient in everyday situations. To assess carryover, ask the caregiver to keep a journal of the patient's functional use of conversations in activities of daily living for your review.

References

Davis, G. A. (2000). *Aphasiology: Disorders and clinical practice.* Needham Heights, MA: Allyn & Bacon.

Gleason, J. B., Goodglass, H., Green, E., Ackerman, N., & Hyde, M. R. (1975). The retrieval of syntax in Broca's aphasia. *Brain and Language, 2,* 451–471.

Helm-Estabrooks, N., & Albert, M. (2004). *Manual of aphasia and aphasia therapy* (2nd ed.). Austin, TX: Pro-Ed.

Helm-Estabrooks, N., & Nicholas, M. (2000). *Sentence production program for aphasia.* Austin, TX: Pro-Ed.

Menn, L., Ramsberger, G., & Helm-Estabrooks, N. (1994). A linguistic communication measure for aphasic narratives. *Aphasiology, 8,* 343–359.

Visual Action Therapy (VAT)

Background

Visual Action Therapy (VAT) is a nonverbal therapeutic approach, which is appropriate for patients with severe impairment (i.e., global aphasia). Patients are trained to generate and produce hand/arm gestures that represent objects. The intent is to ultimately improve the patient's functional communication. (Helm-Estabrooks & Albert, 2004). For example, if a patient is thirsty, he or she will produce a gesture that represents drinking from a cup. VAT takes advantage of preserved skills, such as nonlinguistic, visuospatial and memory skills, and the ability to spontaneously use over-learned gestures. The patient's motivation

and ability to attend to tasks will assist in a successful response to intervention.

This particular treatment program utilizes "alternate symbol systems" (Helm-Estabrooks & Albert, 2004) Researchers discovered that patients with global aphasia still had intact abilities to conceptualize (Gardner et al., 1976). For some of these patients, they had the cognitive abilities needed to produce language which led Helm and Benson (1978) to create the initial VAT program. Helm-Estabrooks et al. (1989), found that it was easier for patients to produce proximal gestures (hand and arm movements) prior to distal gestures (hand-finger movements). The initial program was thereby revised to include a new hierarchy of phases which are discussed in the following.

Treatment Phases

There are three phases to the VAT treatment program: proximal limb VAT (hand-arm movements, such as motor activity of sawing), distal limb VAT (hand-finger movements, such as turning a screwdriver), and oral VAT such as blowing. The stimuli used for all three phases include real objects, line drawings, and action pictures of a figure using the object. The patient moves sequentially through a hierarchy of nine steps that progress from simple (matching objects to pictures) to complex (using gestures to represent hidden objects). The clinician tracks ongoing progress to determine if the patient is ready to progress to the next level or phase (Helm-Estabrooks & Albert, 2004). The nine steps are as follows and proceed in a hierarchical progression from 1–9: (1) matching pictures and objects; (2) object use training; (3) action picture demonstration; (4) following action picture commands; (5) pantomimed gesture demonstration; (6) pantomimed gesture recognition; (7) pantomimed gesture production; (8) representation of hidden objects demonstration; and (9) production of gestures for hidden objects.

Preparation for Training

Clinicians will need:

1. 15 real objects (toys do not count)
2. Shaded line drawings of those objects

3. Action pictures of a simple figure using those objects

Suggestions for proximal limb gestures may include motions used to represent paint stick, gavel, saw, and iron. Distal limb gestures may include motions using a screwdriver, teaspoon, telephone, artist's fine paintbrush, and tea bag, etc. For oral gestures motions may involve postures to indicate a whistle, flower, lollipop, and straw, plus others. For a complete overview of the nine steps of VAT, see Helm-Estabrooks and Albert (2004).

Measuring Outcomes

Pre- and post-VAT measurements are suggested. The Boston Assessment of Severe Aphasia (Helm-Estabrooks, Ramsberger, Nicholas, & Morgan, 1989); and the Nonvocal Communication Scale (NCS) (Borod, Fitzpatrick, Helm-Estabrooks, & Goodglass, 1989) have been used pre and post-VAT. The clinician can also use the Communication Questionnaire which has two components, Expressing Self, and Understanding Information (Helm-Estabrooks, 1996).

VAT Follow-Up Treatment. Helm-Estabrooks and Albert (2004) suggest several steps following successful outcome of VAT:

1. The Amer-Ind Code program, which has been modified by Skelly (1979) for patients with aphasia is based on Native American hand signals. Thirty additional gestures are taught. Such gestures may be used to communicate functional needs, such as "bathroom" and "sleep."
   Refer to Rao (1994) for a recent review of this method.
2. Promoting Aphasics' Communicative Effectiveness (PACE) (Davis & Wilcox, 1981; Helm-Estabrooks & Albert, 2004) suggest using the PACE photo cards to teach two-gesture combinations, such as "man drinking."
3. To ease some of the patient's burden of communication, a family member or other communication partner may be brought into the therapy sessions. The patient is first shown an illustration of an object or concept that is new. They are then asked to use a gesture to communicate

the illustration which the family member, must identify. The clinician's job is to monitor and review progress, so the patient and their communication partner are able to identify areas of weakness that still need improvement. This can be accomplished by carefully charting data or videotaping sessions and reviewing them with both communication partners.

References

Beeson, P. M., Hirsch, F. M., & Rewega, M. A. (2002). Successful single-word writing treatment: Experimental analyses of fours cases. *Aphasiology, 16,* 473–491.

Borod, J., Fitzpatrick, R., Helm-Estabrooks, N., & Goodglass, H. (1989). The relationship between limb apraxia and the spontaneous use of communicative gesture in aphasia. *Brain and Cognition, 10,* 121–131.

Davis, G. A., & Wilcox, M. J. (1981). Incorporating parameters of natural conversation in aphasia treatment. In R. Chapey (Ed.), *Language intervention strategies in adult aphasia.* Baltimore: Lippincott Williams & Wilkins.

Edelman, G. (1987). *P.A.C.E.: Promoting Aphasics' Communicative Effectiveness.* Bicester, England: Winslow Press.

Gardner, H., Zurif, E. B., Berry, T., & Baker, E. H. (1976). Visual communication in aphasia. *Neuropsychologia, 14,* 275–292.

Helm, N. A., & Benson, D. F. (1978). *Visual Action Therapy for global aphasia.* Paper presented at the annual meeting of the Academy of Aphasia, Chicago.

Helm-Estabrooks, N., & Albert, M. L. (2004). The communication questionnaire. *Manual of aphasia and aphasia therapy* (2nd ed. , pp. 188–189). Austin, TX: Pro-Ed.

Helm-Estabrooks, N., & Albert, M. (2004). *Manual of aphasia and aphasia therapy* (2nd ed.). Austin, TX: Pro-Ed (http://proedinc.com).

Helm-Estabrooks, N., Ramsberger, G., Brownell, H., & Albert, M. (1989). Distal versus proximal movement in limb apraxia [Abstract]. *Journal of Clinical and Experimental Neuropsychology, 7,* 608.

Helm-Estabrooks, N., Ramsberger, G., Nicholas, M., & Morgan, A. (1989). *Boston assessment of severe aphasia.* Austin, TX: Pro-Ed.

Rao, P. R. (1994). Use of Amer-Ind Code by persons with aphasia. In R. Chapey (Ed.), *Language intervention strategies in adult aphasia* (pp. 359–367). Baltimore: Williams & Wilkins.

Skelly, M. (1979). *Amer-Ind gestural code based on universal American Indian hand talk.* New York: Elsevier.

INDEX